"Larry Newman and Mo Levin are two of the most gifted teachers and clinicians in the field of headache medicine. . . . *Headache and Facial Pain* is a perfect addition to the series *What Do I Do Now?*, a question many of us ask in the day-to-day practice of our craft. . . . We owe a debt of gratitude to Doctors Newman and Levin for sharing their considerable talents and clinical expertise to a wide range of headache related problems in clinical practice. Keep it on your desk!"

—*Fred Sheftell, MD, Director and Founder New England Center for Headache, Stamford, CT, and Departments of Neurology and Psychiatry and Behavioral Sciences, Albert Einstein College of Medicine, Bronx, NY*

"Headache specialists are in short supply, so most doctors don't have the luxury of consulting one for tricky cases. This book is the next best thing to a curbside consult with a headache expert. Each of the 33 chapters covers a difficult or perplexing headache problem. The vignettes are short, snappy, and evocative, and the ensuing case discussions are frank and clear. . . . The real value of this book is that the cases aren't straightforward and simple. The authors do not shy away from controversy, but instead provide cases that are an authentic reflection of real-life headache practice. For many of the complex problems discussed, evidence about the best course of action is lacking, but treatment decisions must nonetheless be made. In these situations, there is no substitute for expert clinical judgment; this book provides it in abundance. The approach to complex cases for which there isn't a 'right answer' is refreshingly sensible and thoughtful."

—*Elizabeth Loder, MD, MPH, Chief, Division of Headache and Pain, Department of Neurology, Brigham and Women's Hospital, Associate Professor of Neurology, Harvard Medical School, Boston, MA*

"The book is loaded with diagnostic and treatment pearls and, as such, is ideal for trainees and clinicians at all levels who care for patients with headache and facial pain. While the authors saw the need for a quick reference tool, what they produced is an effortless, enjoyable, and educational read that clinicians will spend more than just a few minutes of their time with."

—*David W. Dodick, MD, Professor, Neurology, Mayo Clinic, Phoenix, AZ*

"*Headache and Facial Pain* is filled with wisdom and wit as it provides practical solutions to common problems in the care of headache sufferers."

—*Richard B. Lipton, MD, Professor of Neurology, Director, Montefiore Headache Center, Albert Einstein College of Medicine, New York, NY*

What Do I Do Now?

SERIES CO-EDITORS-IN-CHIEF

Lawrence C. Newman, MD
Director of the Headache Institute
Department of Neurology
St. Luke's-Roosevelt Hospital Center
New York, NY

Morris Levin, MD
Co-director of the Dartmouth Headache Center
Director of the Dartmouth Neurology Residency Training Program
Department of Neurology
Dartmouth Hitchcock Medical Center
Lebanon, NH

Headache
and Facial Pain

Lawrence C. Newman, MD
Director of the Headache Institute
Department of Neurology
St. Luke's-Roosevelt Hospital Center
New York, NY

Morris Levin, MD
Co-director of the Dartmouth Headache Center
Director of the Dartmouth Neurology Residency Training Program
Department of Neurology
Dartmouth Hitchcock Medical Center
Lebanon, NH

OXFORD
UNIVER
2009

OXFORD
UNIVERSITY PRESS

Oxford University Press, Inc., publishes works that further Oxford University's objective of excellence
in research, scholarship, and education.

Oxford New York
Auckland Cape Town Dar es Salaam Hong Kong Karachi
Kuala Lumpur Madrid Melbourne Mexico City Nairobi
New Delhi Shanghai Taipei Toronto

With offices in
Argentina Austria Brazil Chile Czech Republic France Greece
Guatemala Hungary Italy Japan Poland Portugal Singapore
South Korea Switzerland Thailand Turkey Ukraine Vietnam

Published by Oxford University Press, Inc.
198 Madison Avenue, New York, New York 10016
www.oup.com

First issued as an Oxford University Press paperback, 2009

Oxford is a registered trademark of Oxford University Press

Library of Congress Cataloging-in-Publication Data

Newman, Lawrence C., M.D.
Headache and facial pain / Lawrence C. Newman, Morris Levin.
p. ; cm.—(What do I do now?)
Includes bibliographical references and index.
ISBN: 978-0-19-537387-5
1. Headache—Case studies.   2. Facial pain—Case studies. I. Levin, Morris, 1955- II. Title.
III. Series. [DNLM: 1. Headache—therapy.   2. Facial Pain—diagnosis.   3. Facial Pain—therapy.
4. Headache—diagnosis.   5. Headache Disorders—diagnosis.   6. Headache Disorders—therapy.
WL 342 N553h 2009]

RC392.N49 2009   616.8'491—dc22
2008014057

The science of medicine is a rapidly changing field. As new research and clinical experience broaden our
knowledge, changes in treatment and drug therapy occur. The author and publisher of this work have checked
with sources believed to be reliable in their efforts to provide information that is accurate and complete, and in
accordance with the standards accepted at the time of publication. However, in light of the possibility of human
error or changes in the practice of medicine, neither the author, nor the publisher, nor any other party who has
been involved in the preparation or publication of this work warrants that the information contained herein
is in every respect accurate or complete. Readers are encouraged to confirm the information contained herein
with other reliable sources, and are strongly advised to check the product information sheet provided by the
pharmaceutical company for each drug they plan to administer.

9 8 7 6 5 4 3 2 1

Printed in the United States of America
on acid-free paper

This book is dedicated to:

My wife Leslie and my sons Daniel and Eric, who have had to deal with my long hours away from home and my working while at home. Their support and love never wavered even as I know they were thinking, "What is he doing now?"

My parents Kenneth and Elinore, who instilled in me the knowledge that anything is possible if you work hard and who were always there to guide me when I was unsure of "What should I do next?"

My mentors, Drs. Seymour Solomon and Richard Lipton, who always had the time, patience, and knowledge to teach me whenever I asked them "What do I do now?"

Dr. Christine Lay, with whom I have been fortunate to practice headache medicine over the past decade. Thank you for your honesty, professionalism, and friendship. I know whatever you do next will be extraordinary.

—LN

To my wife, Karen—thanks again for your support and love—and to my patients, students, residents, fellows, and mentors over the years.

—ML

Acknowledgments

To bring this volume to completion, a number of things had to happen. First, we had to find a publisher interested in the idea. Then, we had to decide upon a format—one that would work best to achieve the goal we set—to provide clinicians with a helpful tool for answering common diagnostic and treatment questions about headache disorders. Then, we needed to choose a size, shape, and "look" that would serve the same goal. At every step of the way, our editor Craig Panner was enormously helpful and never lost patience with our urge to get things just right. His advice and stewardship were invaluable. Thanks, Craig. Also thanks to David D'Addona and Lynda Crawford for all your help as well.

The writing of these cases and discussions was actually quite enjoyable—thought-provoking, challenging, and satisfying. Having each other to use as a critic for our cases was a huge advantage in the process. So we want to thank each other. Thanks, Mo. Thanks, Larry.

And, of course, thanks to our families. Our wives and children have been particularly patient during the writing of this book. Our patients have been the guiding force in our careers. The primary goal is always to help them feel better. Along the way, they have taught us most of what we know about headache disorders, and we are grateful. Our students at all levels—medical students, residents, and fellows—have been essential in teaching us how best to impart what we have learned to others, and we owe them a debt of gratitude as well.

Finally, to our readers: Thank you for using this book. We hope it helps. We would appreciate feedback (constructive, hopefully, but don't feel constrained).

Lawrence Newman, MD
Morris Levin, MD

Preface

Patients with headache can be among the most challenging in all of medicine. Diagnosis is often perplexing; there are numerous possible tests to choose among and a plethora of treatment options; and there are pitfalls where serious disease lurks. Even experienced clinicians occasionally arrive at the point where diagnostic, work-up, treatment, or prognostic thinking becomes blocked. In short, we all find ourselves from time to time in an exam room or at the bedside, asking ourselves, "What do I do now?" Using standard textbooks or reviewing literature may often be unproductive, and tracking down the correct consultant can be difficult and time-consuming. Having been both consultants and consulters (as well as headache sufferers), we decided there was a need for a quick reference tool that served as a resource for these difficult headache conundrums.

In this book, we have simulated the "curbside consultation" in a representative set of 33 "mini-consultation" scenarios about headache and facial pain. The key questions in each are addressed, much as a consultant would do over the phone or in the hallway. We have divided this volume into three sections that cover the typical ground for head/face pain consultation: (1) Diagnostic Questions, (2) Treatment Considerations, and (3) Prognostic, Social and Legal Issues. Recommendations are based on the most current evidence available. Diagnostic thinking is presented along the lines of the *International Classification of Headache Disorders*, second edition (ICHD-II), which can be found at www.i-h-s.org. A list of key clinical points appears at the end of each case discussion, followed by a list of suggested articles or chapters for those interested in doing further reading on the subject. Tables are provided for quick reference in most chapters.

This book is designed as a resource for clinicians at all levels of training in all fields of medicine who treat patients with headache and facial pain syndromes. We believe it will help to illuminate the aspect of our work most of us entered medical life to pursue – the intellectual challenge of sorting through complex important clinical problems.

LN, New York, NY
ML, Hanover, NH

Contents

brainstem near the trigeminal nuclei. Both diagnostic and treatment approaches (medical and surgical) are discussed in this chapter.

20 Emergency Department and Inpatient Management   98

This chapter reviews the treatment of headache in the emergency department and the indications for inpatient admission. In addition, a variety of treatment strategies are discussed, and tapering methods for butalbital-containing medications and opioids are provided.

21 Occipital Neuralgia   104

Occipital neuralgia (ON) presents with lancinating (often mixed with more aching) occipital pain, which can be very disabling. There are a number of conditions which present, like ON, with posterior pain; but tenderness of the greater occipital nerve and response to greater occipital nerve anesthetic blockade are essentially pathognomonic.

22 Headache Recurrence   109

Recurrence of headache following initially successful treatment occurs in approximately 20% of patients who use triptans for acute relief. This chapter outlines the clinical features of recurrence and provides strategies to avoid it.

23 Headache and Allergy   112

Many patients feel that environmental and dietary allergens or other agents (including additives in medications) can cause them to experience headache. This chapter outlines a reasonable approach to the investigation of dietary and environmental triggers of migraine and other headaches, as well as nonpharmaceutical approaches to pain relief.

24 Headache Treatment in Human Immunodeficiency Virus Infection (HIV) and Drug Addiction   116

Headaches in patients with active HIV infection may stem from a number of causes, including primary headaches unrelated to HIV. Diagnostic approaches are outlined. This chapter also discusses the pitfalls encountered in headache and pain management when treating patients with substance abuse.

25 Pseudotumor   120

Pseudotumor cerebri, or idiopathic intracranial hypertension, often affects young obese women. Hallmarks are headaches of various types, papilledema, and increased opening pressure on lumbar puncture. When headaches or visual dysfunction fail to respond to acetazolamide, there are several other alternatives, which are explained in this chapter.

SECTION III PROGNOSTIC, SOCIAL, AND LEGAL ISSUES

Diagnostic Questions

1 Orgasmic Headaches

A 32-year-old man with a history of occasional moderate headaches, usually occurring during times of stress, describes a new type of headache. It is severe and bifrontal and occurs abruptly only at or near the time of orgasm. There have been approximately 10–12 of these. These do not occur with any other activity and have been so severe as to induce him to abstain from sex. He has been tried unsuccessfully on beta-blocker prophylaxis. Computed tomography (CT) of the head has been normal. His wife is scared that he has an aneurysm since his father "died from one." The headaches have led to marital discord.

What do you do now?

Severe abrupt headaches occurring with exertion are suggestive of subarachnoid hemorrhage (SAH), other intracranial hemorrhage, or arterial dissection. As such, they must be aggressively worked up. Recurring exertional or sex-induced headaches, as in this case, paint a different, more benign picture—in general (See Table 1–1). The imperative is still to rule out serious causes of sudden or "thunderclap headache" (see Table 1–2), including ruptured berry aneurysm, intracranial hemorrhage, cervical arterial dissection, and cerebral venous thrombosis (CVT).

Aneurysmal SAH can easily occur without neurological signs initially, so CT of the head and lumbar puncture are essential. If some time has passed, diagnosis is, of course, more challenging. Intracranial hemorrhage, particularly if small, may also present rather benignly; but neuroimaging is generally unambiguous. Without a magnetic resonance (MR) venogram, CVT may be missed. Assessment by MR angiography (MRA) of the carotids and vertebral arteries will generally exclude it. Another entity that can present rather deceptively is reversible cerebral vasoconstriction syndrome (RCVS), also known as "Call-Fleming syndrome." This generally presents as sudden or severe headache and later with neurological deficits due to ischemic brain injury. Unlike central nervous system vasculitis, the cerebrospinal fluid in RCVS is generally normal and MR imaging (MRI) is often normal as well. The hallmark is the finding of segmental arterial narrowing seen on angiography (see Chapter 10).

TABLE 1-1 **Exertional and Sexual Headaches**

Type	Characteristics
Primary cough headache	Bilateral, severe, short headaches brought on by any Valsalva (important to exclude skull base lesion including Chiari malformation)
Primary exertional headache	Unilateral or bilateral, emerges during exercise, usually in young males
Preorgasmic headache	Dull ache in head/neck/jaw, increasing with sexual excitement
Orgasmic headache	Severe and explosive, frontal or occipital, occurring at or near the time of orgasm
Positional sexual headache	Suboccipital, following intercourse, worse with upright position (thought to be due to dural cerebrospinal fluid leak)

So, how aggressively must the work-up be here? Given the recurring, virtually pathognomonic, nature of these headaches, it is tempting to fit them neatly into the category of the orgasmic headache defined in the *International Classification of Headache Disorders* as "sudden severe headaches occurring at the time of orgasm." A brain MRI to rule out recent hemorrhage, MRA of the cerebral vessels to investigate for aneurysm and segmental narrowing, MRA of the cervical vessels to look for dissection, and an MR venogram to rule out CVT would be a very thorough approach. But is this even enough? When a family member has known berry aneurysm(s), the chance of an aneurysm in an individual may be as much as four times greater than the average risk (general prevalence of cerebral aneurysms is 1%–5%), although this is not entirely clear as some studies only show increased risk of SAH if two immediate family members have had SAH. The question of aneurysm screening commonly comes up even in patients without headaches, so in the case above this is even more pressing. And MRA may not be as sensitive as the patient would like. For many of these cases, CT angiography is providing the answer and could be done here. But now we are up to five expensive neuroimaging investigations.

A parsimonious diagnostic approach to this case could be done in steps, as follows:

1. Thorough neurological examination, including fundoscopy, reveals no deficits.
2. Brain MRI reveals no abnormalities.
3. Treatment leads to adequate resolution of the headaches.

Later, questions of screening for aneurysm in a first-degree relative can be discussed, and close observation for new clues can continue. If treatment proves inadequate, further work-up will be done.

Treatment options for orgasmic head are reasonably good. Indomethacin 25–50 mg about 1 hour prior to intercourse is often successful at completely preventing an attack. Beta-blockers such as propranolol, atenolol, and metoprolol can be effective in case prophylaxis makes more sense (frequency, convenience). A relative contraindication is the possibility of impotence due to these drugs, which can further worsen the marital problems already surfacing. Calcium channel blockers have also been tried. Altering sexual positions has been reported to help.

TABLE 1-2   Causes of Sudden (Thunderclap) Headache

- Subarachnoid hemorrhage or "aneurysmal leak" (sentinel headache)
- Hypertensive, lobar, or pituitary intracranial hemorrhage
- Cerebral venous thrombosis
- Carotid or vertebral artery dissection
- Intracranial hypotension
- Central nervous system vasculitis
- Reversible cerebral vasoconstriction syndrome (RCVS)
- Acute hypertension
- Primary thunderclap headache
- Sphenoid sinusitis
- Colloid cyst of the third ventricle

KEY POINTS TO REMEMBER

- Exertional and sexual headaches can occur as benign primary headaches, but their presentations may indicate underlying structural disease.
- *Thunderclap headache*–a sudden severe headache of any type–may also indicate underlying vascular or other organic pathology, including cerebral aneurysm, cerebral venous thrombosis, and reversible cerebral vasoconstriction syndrome.
- When a family member has known berry aneurysm(s), the chance of an aneurysm in an individual may be as much as four times greater than the average risk.
- As is true for several primary headache disorders, primary orgasmic headache seems to be particularly responsive to indomethacin.

Further Reading

Dodick DW. Thunderclap headache. Curr Pain Headache Rep 2002;6:226-232.

Frese A, Eikermann A, Frese K, et al. Headache associated with sexual activity: demography, clinical features, and comorbidity. Neurology 2003;61:796-800.

Levin M. Exertional headaches. In: Levin M, Ward TN (eds), Head, Neck and Facial Pain. Columbus, OH: Anadem, 2006.

Ronkainen A, Miettinen H, Karkola K, et al. Risk of harboring an unruptured intracranial aneurysm. Stroke 1998;29:359-362.

Sinus Headache

A 45-year-old park ranger has had frequent severe frontal "sinus" headaches for several years, some of which are accompanied by nasal discharge. They are often worsened by bending forward. He develops some nausea with the most severe ones, as well as some photophobia. Antibiotic courses have helped on occasion, but headaches tend to return once the treatment ends. Triptans have been of some use, but he is using frequent over-the-counter (OTC) medications on most days for pain. Magnetic resonance imaging (MRI) of the head reveals maxillary and sphenoid sinus hyperdensities (see Fig. 2-1).

What do you do now?

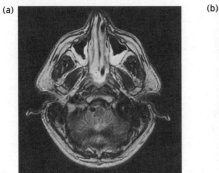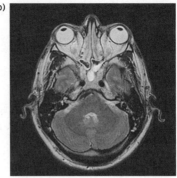

FIGURE 2-1 Bilateral maxillary (a) and sphenoid sinus hyperdensities (b). (Courtesy of John J. McIntyre, MD, Section of Neuroradiology, Dartmouth Hitchcock Medical Center, Lebanon, NH.)

Here, diagnosis is a bit complicated. There are plenty of migraine features (see Table 2–1)—nausea, photophobia, chronicity—but there are also some features suggestive of a nasal or paranasal sinus pain origin—nasal discharge, worsening with dependent position, response to antibiotics (albeit temporary), and the MRI findings. Of course, there is no phonophobia (although it would be worth asking about to make sure), pain is bilateral, and onset is a bit late in life, so the *International Classification of Headache Disorders*, second edition (ICHD II) diagnosis of migraine is far from certain. Also, it is well known that triptans will abort nonmigrainous headaches of many types including even the headache of subarachnoid hemorrhage. At most, one could label this patient's headaches as "probable migraine." So, could this headache be a "sinus headache"?

The ICHD IIR defines headache attributed to rhinosinusitis (11.5, "sinus headache") as headache in the region of the sinuses plus clear clinical, endoscopic, and/or imaging evidence of infection close in timing to the onset of headaches, as well as remission of the pain after sinusitis treatment (Table 2–2).

Thus, using these criteria, one could diagnose "sinus headache" in this case. But why do headaches keep returning? Could the daily use of OTC medications be exacerbating an underlying migraine physiology? The confounding issue, of course, is the high prevalence of both primary headache disorders and sinus-type symptoms in the general population. Many patients self-diagnose sinus headaches, which leads to much overuse of sinus

TABLE 2-1   **ICHD-IIR Diagnostic Criteria for Migraine without Aura**

A. At least five attacks fulfilling criteria B–D
B. Headache attacks lasting 4–72 hours (untreated or successfully treated)
C. Headache has at least two of the following characteristics:
    1. Unilateral location
    2. Pulsating quality
    3. Moderate or severe pain intensity
    4. Aggravation by or causing avoidance of routine physical activity
D. During the headache at least one of the following:
    1. Nausea and/or vomiting
    2. Photophobia and phonophobia
E. Not attributed to another disorder

Source: International Headache Society, *International Classification of Headache Disorders*, second edition. Cephalalgia 2004; 24 (suppl 1): 1–160

TABLE 2-2   **ICHD-IIR Definition of Headache Attributed to Rhinosinusitis**

- Frontal headache accompanied by pain in one or more regions of the face, ears, or teeth
- Clinical, nasal endoscopic, computed tomographic, and/or magnetic resonance imaging and/or laboratory evidence of acute or acute-on-chronic rhinosinusitis
- Headache and facial pain develop simultaneously with onset or acute exacerbation of rhinosinusitis
- Headache and/or facial pain resolve within 7 days after remission or successful treatment of acute or acute-on-chronic rhinosinusitis

remedies. Many physicians likewise are misled by allergy and/or sinus symptoms, leading to overly liberal treatment with antibiotics.

Paranasal sinus imaging has become accurate enough to rule out cases of sinusitis which require surgical and/or medical treatment. When imaging of the nasal and paranasal regions is negative, most clinicians will move on to other possibilities. However, the idea of "chronic sinusitis" or allergy-induced headache (with negative sinus films) is still popular and, we think, generally spurious. (Allergy-related headache is discussed in Chapter 23). When sinus imaging is positive, things are not so straightforward. Does a maxillary polyp hold significance in patients with primary headache? Probably not. What about "mucosal changes"? Again, probably not important. Key imaging findings suggesting sinus pathology which needs further investigation include the following: tissue changes filling one or more sinus cavities; air–fluid levels in maxillary, ethmoid, frontal or sphenoid sinuses; or evidence of bony or other tissue deformity. The best approach in some of these cases, particularly those unresponsive to antibiotics, is to enlist the aid of a skilled otolaryngologist. Endoscopic evaluation and biopsy of sinus tissue is possible, and fungal, parasitic, or resistant/unusual bacterial infections have been discovered in this way.

In the case above, it is crucial to try noninvasive measures aimed at migraine, medication overuse headache, and improving sinus hygiene. The sphenoid sinus opacification is of concern but not crucially so, particularly if repeat imaging shows no further changes. Prophylactic medication for migraine such as beta-blocker, cyclic antidepressant, or anticonvulsive-type medication might be considered discontinuing OTC medication should certainly be encouraged, as should nasal/sinus irrigation and a thorough search for allergic triggers. If these measures fail, endoscopic evaluation seems sensible, including biopsy, in the hope of finding a treatable cause for the sinus-related component of the patient's headaches.

On a more controversial plane, there are a number of otolaryngological conditions which are thought by some to cause headache. These include (1) *concha bullosa* (an expanded turbinate with an air cell in it), (2) nasal septal deviation, (3) *septal spurs* (sharp, bony projections off the septum that can impinge on the lateral nasal wall tissues), and (4) *rhinolithiasis* (foreign bodies trapped in a sinus). The close impingement of mucosal sinus tissues ("contact points") caused by these processes may cause stimulation of nasal branches of the maxillary nerve, leading to local and referred head pain.

KEY POINTS TO REMEMBER

- When patients present with "sinus headaches" as well as some migraine features, it is always best to follow the trails of both, with work-up and treatment aimed at all diagnoses discovered.
- Imaging findings suggestive of sinus-related headaches include filling opacity in one or more sinus cavities; air-fluid levels in maxillary, ethmoid, frontal, or sphenoid sinuses; and evidence of bony changes involving the surrounding osseous structures.
- Endoscopic evaluation, including biopsy, can be diagnostic if noninvasive measures fail.

Further Reading

Cady RK, Schreiber CP. Sinus headache or migraine? Considerations in making a
differential diagnosis. Neurology 2002;58:S10-S14.

Eross E, Dodick DW, Eross M. The Sinus, Allergy and Migraine Study (SAMS). Headache
2007;47:213-224.

Mehle ME, Kremer PS. Sinus CT scan findings in "sinus headache" migraineurs. Headache
2008;48:67-71.

3 White Matter Abnormalities on Magnetic Resonance Imaging

A 37-year-old woman presents with bilateral, throbbing headaches associated with nausea and photophobia. Headaches occur three times monthly and respond to treatment with non-steroidal anti-inflammatory drugs. Her maternal grandmother suffered from migraine without aura. She reports right arm numbness accompanying some of her headaches as well as increasing frequency of headaches over the last several months. The patient's medical and neurological examinations are normal. Because of these new symptoms, you order magnetic resonance imaging (MRI) of the brain, which reveals scattered white matter hyperintensities on T2 (Fig. 3-1). The radiologist's report states that demyelinating disease must be excluded.

What do you do now?

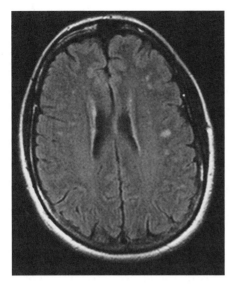

FIGURE 3-1 Typical white matter lesions of migraine on magnetic resonance imaging.

White matter hyperintensities (WMH) are a common incidental finding on brain MRI, occurring in approximately 10% of people aged 30–40 years. The prevalence of WMH increases with age, and they are also seen more commonly in individuals with hypertension, diabetes, hypercholesterolemia, cerebrovascular and cardiovascular disease, multiple sclerosis (MS), and collagen vascular and other autoimmune disorders. Because the causes of WMH are so extensive, determining their etiology can at times be difficult.

Although most migraine sufferers have normal MRIs, the most common MRI abnormality in migraineurs is WMH. The prevalence of WMH in migraine ranges 12%–46%. These abnormalities are usually characterized by small, multiple, punctate hyperintensities that are best seen on both T2-weighted and fluid attenuation inversion recovery (FLAIR) sequences. The WMH of migraine are typically bilateral and most often located in the deep white matter, but the localization in migraine varies with age. Prior to age 40, migraineurs are more likely to have these WMH in the centrum semiovale and frontal subcortical white matter. After age 40, the lesions are predominantly localized in the deeper white matter, at the level of the basal ganglia.

Migraine sufferers are four times more likely than nonmigraineurs to have WMH on MRI. This increased risk is independent of age and vascular risk factors. Although there does not appear to be an association between the presence or severity of periventricular WMH and migraine, there is a twofold risk for lesions in the deep white matter in women with migraine. This risk is highest in women who suffer from more than one migraine monthly.

The cause of the WMH in migraine is not known. In general, hyperintensities in these areas are thought to be the result of ischemic damage or demyelination, so either of these processes may occur in migraine. It has been postulated that the WMH that occur in migraine may be secondary to abnormal platelet aggregation with subsequent microemboli, hypoperfusion states that occur during aura, or cerebrovascular dysregulation. Perhaps focal hypermetabolic phenomena occur during migraine, leading to an "outstripping" of the blood supply, resulting in focal ischemic injuries.

Among the myriad causes of WMH, those that occur with headaches as a significant manifestation include migraine with and without aura, mitochondrial encephalopathy with lactic acidosis and stroke-like episodes (MELAS), cerebral autosomal dominant arteriopathy with subcortical infarcts and leukoencephalopathy (CADASIL), central nervous system vasculitis, systemic vasculitides that involve cerebral arteries, anticardiolipin antibody syndrome, and MS. The WMH is these disorders differ in their location, appearance, and numbers. The WMH of CADASIL are symmetrical and confluent and are best visualized on T2 and FLAIR sequences. These WMH are most prominent in the frontal and anterior temporal lobes and are associated with diffuse lacunar-type infarcts in the deep white matter and basal ganglia. The MRI changes in MELAS have a predilection for the occipital and temporal lobes and involve both the gray and white matter. The MRI lesions in vasculitis also affect the gray and white matter, and the WMH tend to be contrast-enhancing. The hyperintensities in MS resemble those seen in migraine but, unlike migraine, involve the corpus callosum, cerebellum, and brainstem. The appearance of the periventricular WMH in MS differs as well. Rather than the small, punctate findings of migraine, MS produces ovoid lesions that align perpendicularly to the ventricles ("Dawson's fingers").

The absence of a family history of recurrent strokes and dementia and only one family member with migraine make CADASIL unlikely in our patient. Similarly, MELAS can be eliminated by the clinical history. A prior history of fetal loss, thrombosis, and thrombocytopenia would be expected in the anticardiolipin syndrome and is not reported by this patient. Migraine-like headaches are reported by many patients with MS, and the new onset of numbness in this young woman together with the abnormalities on her MRI make this a possibility. Indeed, in the early stages of MS, the WMH are quite similar to those seen in migraine (and in this patient). However, the location of the WMH in this case is much more typical for migraine than for MS. Specifically, the MRI demonstrates scattered punctate lesions in the centrum semiovale and frontal regions.

No further investigations are needed for our patient at this time. Her history and MRI findings are characteristic of migraine with aura, and the numbness is almost certainly a sensory aura. However, should her complaints change or her neurological examination become abnormal, she should be reevaluated. At that point, repeat MRI can assess for change in lesion count and location. Lumbar puncture might be appropriate for evaluation of possible demyelinating or inflammatory disease. Evoked potentials can be done to assess for subclinical demyelinating disease.

The other question which often arises is one of management. If these WMH in fact represent some form of ischemic damage, might prophylaxis with aspirin or another platelet antiaggregant medication be reasonable? At least, more careful attention might be devoted to nonpharmaceutical prophylaxis of cerebrovascular disease, such as control of blood pressure and lipid levels. There is no evidence yet to support this, but ongoing research is aimed at finding some answers.

KEY POINTS TO REMEMBER

- White matter hyperintensities are four times more likely than in nonmigraineurs, particularly in women.
- White matter hyperintensities are generally small, punctate lesions, affecting deep white matter and best seen on T2 and FLAIR sequences.
- White matter hyperintensities are more common in frontal subcortical regions and the centrum semiovale before age 40 and in deeper white matter and the basal ganglia after age 40.

Further Reading

De Benedittis G, Lorenzetti A, Sina C, et al. Magnetic resonance imaging in migraine and tension-type headache. Headache 1995;36:246-248.

Fazekas F. Magnetic resonance signal abnormalities in asymptomatic individuals: their incidence and functional correlates. Eur Neurol 1989;29:865-885.

Igarashi H, Sakai F, Kan S, et al. Magnetic resonance imaging in patients with migraine. Cephalalgia 1991;11:69-74.

Kruit MC, van Buchem MA, Hofman PA, et al. Migraine as a risk factor for subclinical brain lesions. JAMA 2004;291:427-434.

Osborn RE, Alder DC, Mitchell CS. MR imaging of the brain in patients with migraine headaches. Am J Neuroradiol 1991;12:521-524.

Porter A, Gladstone JP, Dodick DW. Migraine and white matter hyperintensities. Curr Headache Rep 2005;4:141-145.

Soges LJ, Cacayorin ED, Petro GR, et al. Migraine: evaluation by MR. Am J Neuroradiol 1988;9:425-429.

4 Childhood Migraine

A 10-year-old, 30 kg boy has had severe unilateral throbbing headaches for the past 2 years. They are accompanied by nausea and vomiting, photophobia, phonophobia, and fatigue. Headaches occur approximately once per month but can occur more frequently during hot weather and with stress (e.g., around the time his parents were contemplating divorce). His headaches are dramatically responsive to zolmitriptan 5 mg, although he experiences a 20-minute period of very bothersome aching pain and tension in his jaw and neck. He is now all out of zolmitriptan.

What do you do now?

This child almost certainly has migraine. The diagnosis of migraine in children is a bit challenging since the features may differ from the standard definition in adults. Specifically, the headaches may be shorter, they are commonly bilateral, and auras are rarer. Treatment has typically centered around nonpharmacological measures such as sleep hygiene, regular meal-times, and avoidance of triggers, with the judicious use of analgesics and antiemetics. However, this is not a satisfying approach when the child has very severe headaches which are disabling. School, social, and family activities suffer; and the child can develop secondary psychological consequences (see Chapter 27). Acute treatment and prophylaxis, of course, go hand in hand. A number of prophylactic agents are in common use, although few have a formal Food and Drug Administration (FDA) indication for prevention of migraine in children. Beta-blockers, cyclic antidepressants, calcium channel blockers, and the anticonvulsants divalproex sodium (Depakote) and topiramate (Topamax) have been shown to help some children and adolescents. Cyproheptadine (Periactin) has been advocated for some time as a useful preventive agent as well. These medications have the potential to affect (to varying degrees) energy levels, sleep patterns, and cognition, so careful monitoring of adverse effects must be a high priority.

In the analgesic class, ibuprofen and acetaminophen have the best evidence supporting their use in children. Other non-steroidal anti-inflammatory drugs (NSAIDS), such as naproxen sodium, have been widely used as well. Antiemetics such as promethazine (Phenergan) and metoclopramide (Reglan) can be very effective when used judiciously. Extrapyramidal symptoms related to antiemetic/neuroleptic medication use, including *akathisia* (restlessness) and *dystonia* (muscular spasms of the neck, eyes, tongue, or jaw), are more common in children than adults, so close observation is indicated.

As for triptans, none has gained FDA approval for use in children (or even adolescents). Of the eight triptan-containing formulations now on the market, sumatriptan, rizatriptan, naratriptan, eletriptan, and zolmitriptan have been studied in children. These studies were done with small populations and led to generally positive results, although not conclusive. Billinghurst et al. (2004) did a meta-analysis of all the studies done up to 2004 and found the most encouraging results with sumatriptan. Clinical experience in headache clinics, however, seems to offer much more support for the use of nearly all of the triptans in children, with relatively little in the way of adverse effects to worry about. Serious triptan complications related to hypertension and vascular constriction seem to be virtually nonexistent in children, as might be expected. (The risks are probably overrated in adults as well according to most researchers.) Children do experience the less serious, but still troublesome, adverse effects seen in the general population, such as jaw tightness and other muscular symptoms, sensation changes, sedation, and nausea (Table 4–1). They may also experience central nervous system side effects, which can interfere with school performance. One of the features of the triptans most written about is the fact that their effects differ among users. This is sometimes so marked as to prompt the trial of multiple triptans in patients to find the most effective and least offensive agent.

In the case above, there are really two steps which should be taken. First, the safety of triptans should not be taken entirely for granted. A thorough physical exam should be given to make sure cardiovascular and other systems are normal. Since the features of this boy's headaches are so suggestive of migraine, neuroimaging is probably not essential, particularly if there is a strong family history. Of course, full neurological and head and neck exams must be done, and diagnostic decision making should always be discussed fully with the parents. Second, if no contraindications are found to the use of triptans, an alternative triptan might be tried in the hope of avoiding the annoying jaw and neck tightness. Perhaps almotriptan (Axert) or naratriptan (Amerge) could be tried as adverse effects seem lower with these two. Doses are not clearly known but half of the usual adult dose would seem reasonable given this patient's weight.

Another thought is to try an NSAID or even a combination medication such as Midrin, composed of isometheptene mucate (a sympathomimetic

TABLE 4-1 Common Triptan Side Effects

- Dizziness, light-headedness
- Paresthesias, hot or cold sensations
- Nausea
- Muscular pain and tightness
- Dry mouth
- Chest pain (generally noncardiac)

amine), dichloralphenazone (a mild sedative), and acetaminophen. Opioid analgesics can sometimes be useful too, although exacerbation of nausea and risk of habituation are important issues. Again, parental involvement is important since none of these acute medications has been shown to be effective and completely safe in children. (See Table 4–2 for a list of acute medications used in treating migraine in children.)

TABLE 4-2 **Acute Medications Used in Treating Migraine in Children. (Typical doses for children >40 kg in weight are shown although evidence for effectiveness and tolerance is incomplete)**

Medication	Typical Dose
Ibuprofen	200-800 mg or 5-10 mg/kg
Acetaminophen	325-650 mg or 10 mg/kg
Isometheptene mucate (Midrin)	1-2 capsules at onset
Acetaminophen with codeine	300 mg + 30 mg po
Sumatriptan	25-50 mg po or 5 mg nasal
Almotriptan	6.5 mg po
Zolmitriptan	2.5 mg po
Rizatriptan	5 mg po
Naratriptan	1.25-2.5 mg po
Eletriptan	20-40 mg po
Promethazine (Phenergan)	12.5 mg suppository, 25 mg po (for nausea)
Metoclopramide (Reglan)	5 mg po (for nausea)

KEY POINTS TO REMEMBER

- Migraine in children differs from the adult form in several ways: (1) the headache can be shorter; (2) unilaterality is less common, as are auras; and (3) lifestyle adjustment can be very helpful.
- While triptans are not approved for use in children (or adolescents), judicious use with open discussion with parents is common practice.
- Both acute medications and prophylactic agents may produce significant adverse effects in children that must be monitored closely.

Further Reading

Billinghurst L, Richer L, Russell K, et al. Systematic review of acute migraine therapy in children. Headache 2004;44:464-465.

Damen L, Bruijn JKJ, Verhagen AP, et al. Symptomatic treatment of migraine in children: a systematic review of medication trials. Pediatrics 2005;116;e295-e302.

Dodick DW, Martin V. Triptans and CNS side effects. Cephalalgia 2004;24:417-424.

Dodick DW, Martin VT, Smith T, Silberstein S. Cardiovascular tolerability and safety of triptans: a review of clinical data. Headache 2004;44(suppl 1):S20-S30.

Gladstein J. Triptans in children and adolescents. Drug Dev Res 2007;68:346-349.

5 Giant Cell Arteritis

A 78-year-old woman complains of 2 weeks of severe left-sided headaches. She reports body aches, fatigue, and pain on combing her hair. Her exam reveals a hardened left temporal artery. Her sedimentation rate is 120 mm/hour, C-reactive protein is 2.5 mg/dL, and biopsy is negative despite multiple sections and bilateral biopsy. She is a brittle diabetic on insulin.

What do you do now?

With this case the clinician faces a dilemma. Failure to treat a patient with giant cell arteritis (GCA) portends devastating consequences, yet so too does needlessly exposing a brittle diabetic to the effects of long-term steroid use. The most common primary vasculitis in adulthood, GCA affects medium and large arteries. This inflammatory arteritis has its onset almost always after age 50 years, and the highest incidence occurs in the seventh and eighth decades of life. It affects women three times more often than men and occurs more commonly in whites than other races.

Clinically, GCA may present in a variety of ways. A new onset of headache is reported in up to 75% of patients with GCA. These headaches may be associated with constitutional symptoms such as fever, joint and muscle pains, anorexia, weight loss, and fatigue. As many as 40% of patients with GCA also have polymyalgia rheumatica. Additional findings include abnormalities of the temporal artery (beading, prominence, tenderness, pulselessness), jaw claudication, scalp tenderness, tongue or scalp necrosis, diplopia, elevated erythrocyte sedimentation rate (ESR), and visual changes. Indeed, it is the potential for GCA to cause a rapidly sequential, bilateral blindness that makes early recognition and treatment of paramount importance. Vagaries in presentation make this disorder challenging. Although headache is reported by most patients with GCA, it is also common in many other conditions. Jaw claudication, commonly attributed to GCA, is in fact present in only 34% of sufferers. Twenty percent of patients with GCA report no systemic symptoms.

Because GCA can present with a number of different clinical scenarios and because many of the features of GCA are vague and nonspecific, the ability of the clinician to correctly diagnose the syndrome with a high level of sensitivity is a key concern. The American College of Rheumatology diagnostic criteria for GCA are listed in Table 5–1. The presence of three or more of these criteria yields a sensitivity of 93.5% and a specificity of 91.2%. Rodriguez-Valverde and coworkers (1997) developed an alternate set of criteria that combines clinical features and laboratory testing. In these criteria, an age of onset ≥70 years, new-onset headache, and abnormal temporal artery examination have a positive predictive value of 93%. If jaw claudication occurs in addition to the above three criteria, the positive predictive value increases to 100%. Other positive clinical predictors, culled from a meta-analysis of patients with GCA, include, in descending order of

1. Age at onset ≥50 years
2. New-onset or new type of headache
3. Temporal artery tenderness to palpation or decreased pulsation, unrelated to cervical artery arteriosclerosis
4. Erythrocyte sedimentation rate ≥50 mm/hour by Westergren method
5. Abnormal temporal artery biopsy showing vasculitis characterized by a predominance of mononuclear cell infiltration or granulomatous infiltration, usually with multinucleated giant cells

Source: Melson et al. (2007).

likeliness, beading of the temporal artery, prominent or enlarged temporal artery, jaw claudication, diplopia, absent temporal artery pulse, tender temporal artery, or any temporal artery finding.

If GCA is considered likely by clinical history and physical examination, a work-up demonstrating elevations in ESR and C-reactive protein (CRP) should be done. Abnormalities on these tests signal the presence of a systemic inflammatory process and should be corroborated by temporal artery biopsy (TAB). Several clinical factors predict the likelihood of a positive TAB. The likelihood ratio is a direct estimate of how much a test result will change the odds of having a disease. This ratio may be expressed as either a positive or a negative value. The likelihood ratio for a positive result tells you how much the odds of the disease increase when a test is positive. The likelihood ratio for a negative result tells you how much the odds of the disease decrease when a test is negative. The likelihood ratio of a positive TAB in patients with an abnormal ESR is 1.1. As the ESR rises above 50 mm/hour, the likelihood ratio also rises, to 1.2; and when the ESR is >100, the likelihood of a positive biopsy is 1.9. As the ESR may be normal in approximately 17% of patients with GCA, a more useful marker is the CRP level. Elevated CRP was found in 100% of patients with biopsy-proven GCA. The sensitivity of an elevated CRP was reported to be 97.5%, and when both ESR and CRP were elevated, the sensitivity increased to 99%. If clinical suspicion is high, even in the presence of normal inflammatory markers, TAB should be performed since missing the diagnosis of GCA is associated with significant morbidity while the risk of TAB is quite low.

Temporal artery biopsy is considered the gold standard for the diagnosis of GCA, and the yield of a positive biopsy may be optimized by taking a long sample (2–5 cm) from the symptomatic side and instructing the pathologist to examine multiple, thin, serial cuts done at small intervals. This ensures that false-negative results are minimized as GCA may cause "skip" lesions, in which segments of the vessel are affected in a discontinuous pattern. The sensitivity of a unilateral TAB is approximately 90% and is slightly higher for bilateral sections. In general, unilateral TAB is usually sufficient; however, contralateral biopsies may be performed when the first biopsy is normal in a patient in whom there is a high clinical suspicion for GCA. Although the yield of the additional biopsy is seemingly low, averaging approximately 5%, it may uncover the disease in patients with a previously false-negative biopsy.

Our patient meets the American College of Rheumatology criteria for GCA, fulfilling four of the five requirements. Furthermore, using the clinical predictors of GCA established by Smetana and Shmerling (2002), the presence of left temporal artery hardening increased the likelihood that our patient has GCA (positive likelihood ratio of 2), as does her increased ESR >100 (positive likelihood ratio of 1.9). Using the alternative diagnostic criteria of Rodriguez-Valverde et al. (1997), this patient's clinical history gives us a positive predictive value for GCA of 93%.

The overwhelming odds are that this patient does in fact have GCA despite two negative TABs, and a very good case can be made for initiating therapy with steroids. However, in light of the potential serious consequences associated with long-term steroid use, especially in our patient who is a brittle diabetic, perhaps a more prudent approach would be to utilize other diagnostic modalities to confirm the diagnosis. Treatment may be initiated during the expanded investigation and then either discontinued or maintained pending conclusive results. Other laboratory findings associated with GCA include an elevated platelet count, even in the absence of other inflammatory markers.

Thrombocytosis was reported to have a positive likelihood ratio of 6 in predicting that a patient would be diagnosed with GCA. Plasma interleukin-6 elevations have been reported to be present in GCA and can be used as an indicator of active disease. This marker has been reported to be a more accurate gauge of disease activity than the ESR. Fibrinogen levels are also elevated in GCA and may also be a useful indicator of the disease. Because fibrinogen levels are not elevated in other conditions that are associated with high ESR levels, fibrinogen may be a useful marker for the diagnosis, especially in patients with an elevated ESR but few clinical findings.

Other studies that may help in establishing the diagnosis include ultrasonography and magnetic resonance imaging (MRI) of the superficial temporal artery. Color Doppler ultrasonography may reveal a "halo" in the vessel wall, and MRI with contrast may reveal changes in vessel wall thickness and lumen narrowing; but neither study is sensitive or specific enough to supplant TAB. These tests can, however, be used to direct the location for the biopsy. Another option for our patient, and for other patients in whom clinical suspicion for GCA is high despite negative TAB, would be to image the aorta and great vessels via magnetic resonance angiography, positron emission tomography, or conventional angiography. Giant cell arteritis is associated with vasculitis of the aorta and other large vessels and is a risk factor for aneurysms of the abdominal and thoracic portions of the aorta. Imaging of these large vessels in GCA may reveal mural thickening, changes in luminal diameter, or aneurysmal formation.

KEY POINTS TO REMEMBER

- Giant cell arteritis is the most common primary arteritis in patients older than 50 years.
- Giant cell arteritis affects medium and large vessels, including the aorta and its branches.
- Giant cell arteritis can cause a rapidly sequential, bilateral blindness.
- Headache is the most common initial symptom.
- Jaw claudication affects only 34%; 20% have no systemic symptoms.
- The ESR is normal in 17% of patients; CRP is a more sensitive marker.
- Treatment is warranted, even in patients likely to have some degree of intolerance to steroids, when diagnosis is nearly certain.

Further Reading

Hunder GG, Bloch DA, Michel BA, et al. The American College of Rheumatology 1990 criteria for the classification of giant cell arteritis. Arthritis Rheum 1990;33:1122-1128.

Levin M, Ward TN. Horton's disease: past and present. Curr Pain Headache Rep 2005;9:259-266.

Melson MR, Weyand CM, Newman NJ, Biousse V. The diagnosis of giant cell arteritis. Rev Neurol Dis 2007;4:128-142.

Rodriguez-Valverde V, Sarabia JM, Gonzales-Gay MA, et al. Risk factors and predictive models of giant cell arteritis in polymyalgia rheumatica. Am J Med 1997;102:331-336.

Shmerling RH. An 81-year-old woman with temporal arteritis. JAMA 2006;295:2525-2534.

Smetana GW, Shmerling RH. Does this patient have temporal arteritis? JAMA 2002;287:92-101.

Carotid Dissection

You are called to the emergency department to consult on a 29-year-old man without prior headache history who now complains of 2 days of left periorbital throbbing pain, without associated nausea, vomiting, or photo- or phonophobia. His mother and sister suffer from migraine. Exam reveals a left-sided ptosis and miosis. Magnetic resonance imaging (MRI) of the brain and magnetic resonance angiography (MRA) of the head and neck are normal. The patient reports that his head pain was temporarily completely relieved following intravenous dihydroergotamine and metoclopramide when he was seen yesterday in the emergency room and diagnosed with migraine.

What do you do now?

This patient needs to be more thoroughly evaluated. Despite the positive family history, normal imaging, and response to antimigraine therapies, his headaches do not meet the criteria for migraine. Furthermore, the first ever attack of head pain and abnormal findings on his neurological examination strongly suggest a secondary headache disorder (see Table 10–1). Horner syndrome can be seen in cluster headache, but this patient's symptoms are not really consistent with any of the trigeminal autonomic cephalalgias.

Spontaneous dissection of the internal carotid artery is a not uncommon but frequently underrecognized cause of severe headache associated with neurological disturbances in young patients. The annual incidence of spontaneous carotid dissections ranges from 2.5 to 3 per 100,000 and accounts for 5%–20% of strokes in patients younger than 40 years. Dissections most commonly involve the extracranial portion of the artery, and the cervical segment is most often affected. Spontaneous dissections may arise from an underlying arteriopathy resulting from an unidentified connective tissue disorder. Conditions reported to be associated with these spontaneous dissections include Marfan and Behçet syndromes, Ehlers-Danlos type IV, osteogenesis imperfecta type I, fibromuscular dysplasia, and autosomal dominant polycystic kidney disease.

Clinically, carotid dissection may present in a number of ways. Headache is usually the inaugural symptom, occasionally associated with neck pain. The pain usually begins gradually but occasionally presents with a thunderclap onset. Head pain is almost always ipsilateral to the dissection but may be reported to occur as a bifrontal or global headache. Face, ear, and eye pain may accompany the headache; and approximately one-quarter of patients with spontaneous dissections report ipsilateral neck pain. The headaches are usually steady and constant; approximately 25% describe a throbbing quality. Pain severity ranges from mild discomfort to incapacitating.

In a significant minority of patients (45%) the headache of carotid dissection usually precedes the other associated symptoms. Retinal or cerebral ischemia is the most common symptom associated with carotid dissection and may present as visual obscurations and scintillations, amaurosis fugax, transient ischemic attacks, and stroke. Partial Horner syndrome is the most frequent sign of carotid dissection, occurring in as many as 58% of patients. Other associated symptoms include pulsatile tinnitus, syncope, cranial nerve palsies, and dysgeusia.

Although these types of dissections are classified as spontaneous to distinguish them from traumatic dissections, they often follow some "triggering" event. Spontaneous dissections have been reported to occur after vomiting, chiropractic manipulation, sporting events without associated trauma, scuba diving, and going to the hairdresser.

Conventional angiography has long been considered the gold standard for establishing the diagnosis of carotid dissection. Angiographic evidence of dissection is characterized by the presence of a "string sign," a double lumen, or internal flaps. If the dissection involves the subadventitial layer of the vessel so that there is no narrowing of the lumen, angiography may miss the diagnosis. Both MRI and MRA have been demonstrated to be very reliable in diagnosing dissections and are especially useful in diagnosing subadventitial dissections. Helical computed tomography (CT) has also proven to be very sensitive in diagnosing extracranial carotid dissections, as has ultrasonography.

Upon establishing the diagnosis, treatment is aimed at preventing stroke. Most reports suggest that treatment with anticoagulants should begin following diagnosis. Heparin followed by 6 months of oral anticoagulants is the standard treatment, although evidence for this recommendation is considered grade C. Noninvasive monitoring with MRA, CT angiography, and ultrasonography is also recommended.

Our patient had a new-onset headache with an ipsilateral partial Horner syndrome. This painful Horner strongly suggests an extracranial carotid dissection. The negative scans do not rule out dissection. A conventional angiogram should be done and may reveal a dissection of the left carotid artery.

KEY POINTS TO REMEMBER

- Carotid dissection is a not uncommon but frequently underrecognized cause of headache and neurological disturbances in young patients.
- It accounts for 5%–20% of strokes in patients younger than 40 years.
- It most commonly involves the extracranial portion of the artery, and the cervical segment is most often affected.

Continued

- A painful Horner syndrome should suggest the possibility of a silent carotid dissection until proven otherwise.
- Approximately 5% of sufferers have other family members who have had dissections of the aorta or one of its major branches including the carotid.
- Anticoagulation with heparin is recommended for 6 months followed by oral warfarin to prevent carotid thrombosis and embolism.

Further Reading

Baumgartner RW, Arnold M, Baumgartner I, et al. Carotid dissection with and without ischemic events: local symptoms and cerebral artery findings. Neurology 2001;57:827-832.

Mokri B, Sundt TM, Houser OW, Piepgras DG. Spontaneous dissection of the cervical internal carotid artery. Ann Neurol 1986;19:126-138.

Sturzenegger M. Spontaneous internal carotid artery dissection: early diagnosis and management in 44 patients. J Neurol 1995;242:231-238.

Chiari Malformation and Migraine

A 37-year-old man with a long-standing history of headaches suggestive of migraine is seeing you for the first time. He has never sought medical care for his headaches as they are relatively infrequent and until recently responded to over-the-counter products; however, over the past 3 months the headache severity has increased, causing him to miss work. Although his medical and neurological examinations are normal, you order magnetic resonance imaging, which reveals a Chiari malformation type I (CMI) (Fig. 7-1). At his follow-up visit the patient informs you that he has consulted with a neurosurgeon, who recommended surgery. The patient asks for your advice regarding the procedure.

What do you do now?

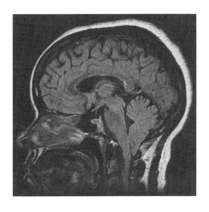

FIGURE 7-1 Chiari malformation. (Courtesy of Gordon Heller, MD, Department of Neuro-Radiology, Roosevelt Hospital Center, New York, NY.)

Chiari malformations are congenital deformities that are thought to arise from intrauterine underdevelopment of the posterior cranial fossa. The resultant crowding of the posterior fossa causes a downward displacement of the cerebellar tonsils through the foramen magnum and into the upper cervical spinal canal. In CMI, the tonsils extend at least 3 mm below the level of the foramen magnum. In CMII, there is descent of the cerebellar tonsils, the cerebellar inferior vermis, and portions of the cerebellar hemispheres into the spinal canal, along with displacement of the brainstem and fourth ventricle. The most frequent form of Chiari malformation is CMII, which is associated with spina bifida and hydrocephalus. Although the exact prevalence of CMI is unknown, it is believed to be a rare disorder, affecting less than 1% of the population, with a slight female predominance.

Many patients with CMI are asymptomatic, and the deformity is discovered incidentally. When symptomatic, clinical features usually present after age 30. Headache is the most common symptom of CMI, although other symptoms can include dizziness, diplopia, dysphagia, nausea, weakness, and ataxia. Pain localization is often occipital–nuchal but may be generalized. Approximately 30% of patients with CMI report headaches that are precipitated by Valsalva maneuvers such as sneezing, laughing, straining, lifting, or bending over; and approximately 20% of CMI patients experience cough headache (see Chapter 13). These cough-induced headaches are characterized by sudden-onset, short-lasting (seconds to minutes), sharp or stabbing pains of moderate to severe intensity, without associated features.

Also, CMI can be associated with headaches that last up to several days and rarely may cause a continuous headache of fluctuating intensity.

It has been postulated that the Valsalva and cough headaches associated with CMI may be the result of transient pressure dissociation between the intracranial and intraspinal compartments that causes the cerebellar tonsils to further extend through the foramen magnum, producing pain via traction and pressure on pain-sensitive structures. The pathophysiological correlates of the other headache subtypes are not known. Some investigators believe that the occipitonuchal headaches are also the result of tonsillar descent (see Pasqual et al, 1992), but others found no relationship between the descent of the tonsils and the presence or absence of headache (see Stovner, 1993).

Our patient is suffering from migraine headaches. He reports no history of occipitonuchal, Valsalva, or cough headaches. The headache of CMI is by definition a secondary headache, and there is no evidence suggesting that this anomaly produces a primary headache disorder. In the various reviews of headache and CMI, the prevalence of migraine and tension-type headaches was similar to that of the general population. Because many CMI patients are asymptomatic, they are identified only when they have a neuroimaging procedure done for another reason. Because migraine is so common, the co-occurrence of the two disorders will occur by chance in many people, as it has in our patient. In these asymptomatic patients there is no indication for a suboccipital craniotomy. Even when patients have headache symptoms consistent with CMI, the indication for suboccipital craniotomy is not clear, although there have been many successes. Complications of surgery include recurrent infection and the formation of fluid accumulations and cysts.

KEY POINTS TO REMEMBER

- Headaches with CMI are the most common symptom.
- Headaches with CMI are usually occipitonuchal.
- Headaches with CMI worsen with Valsalva maneuvers, especially coughing.

Continued

- Headaches with CMI result from transient pressure dissociation between the intracranial and intraspinal compartments, causing increased tonsillar descent through the foramen magnum.
- Headaches with CMI may co-occur in patients with migraine or tension-type headaches but are not causal of these primary headaches.

Further Reading

Meadows J, Kraut M, Guarnieri M, et al. Asymptomatic Chiari type I malformations identified on magnetic resonance imaging. J Neurosurg 2000;92:920–926.

Pascual J, Oterino A, Berciano J. Headache in type I Chiari malformation. Neurology 1992;42:1519–1521.

Riveira C, Pasqual J. Is Chiari type I malformation a reason for chronic daily headache? Curr Pain Headache Rep 2007;11:53–55.

Stovner LJ. Headache associated with the Chiari type I malformation. Headache 1993;33:175–181.

New Daily Persistent Headache

A 24-year-old graduate student is referred by her primary-care physician and a local pain clinic due to unremitting headaches. She is vague as to the nature of the pain and states that the location is "basically all over." She is clear about the onset of pain however: It began on a specific date last summer, the day after an anniversary party for her grandparents when she had some alcohol, talked with many relatives, and slept badly in a small bed. She thinks she also had an upper respiratory virus. At times, she is a bit nauseated by the pain but has not had photo- or phonophobia. Pain is really not triggered or exacerbated by anything, but she is very frustrated at the persistence of the pain and writes as her goal on your intake form "I just want to have a pain-free day." She shows you a list of many migraine prophylactic and acute medications which have not been helpful. Medical history is unremarkable. She is an avid athlete, having been a competitive diver in college. Examination is remarkable for tachycardia at 108 and a fair amount of pain behavior but normal blood pressure and normal neurological examination.

What do you do now?

ew daily persistent headache (NDPH) is a recently identified primary
headache disorder of mysterious origin. The pain is nondescript but
can be severe. Although NDPH is reminiscent of transformed migraine,
there are few migrainous features. It is identical in morphology to the classic
description of chronic tension-type headache but has the unique feature of
starting "out of the blue" for no particular reason (Table 8–1). Virtually
all patients remember almost exactly when the headache started, and the
large majority can name a specific date of onset. Often, patients can recall
a viral-type illness just preceding the onset of the headaches, but this is
not universal. A previous history of headaches is common, as is a family
headache history. There is a female predominance. The patient described
seems to fit the category well, including NDPH's notorious resistance to
treatment.

The most important first step in cases like these is to exclude secondary
causes, particularly treatable ones, such as neoplastic disease, cerebral vasculitis, cerebral venous thrombosis, chronic sinusitis (particularly sphenoid
sinusitis, which may have a paucity of "sinus" symptoms), idiopathic intracranial hypertension (pseudotumor cerebri, which of course may present
without the usual papilledema; see Chapter 25), low cerebrospinal fluid
(CSF) pressure headache syndrome (see Chapter 9), and cervical arterial
or spinal disease. Treatable systemic illness, such as endocrinological disease, chronic infections, or collagen vascular disease, can also lead to daily

TABLE 8-1   **ICHD-II Diagnostic Criteria for New Daily Persistent Headache**

A. Headache that, within 3 days of onset, fulfills criteria B-D

B. Headache is present daily and unremitting for >3 months

C. At least two of the following pain characteristics:
   1. Bilateral location
   2. Pressing/tightening (nonpulsating) quality
   3. Mild or moderate intensity
   4. Not aggravated by routine physical activity such as walking or climbing

D. Both of the following:
   1. No more than one of photophobia, phonophobia, or mild nausea
   2. Neither moderate or severe nausea nor vomiting

E. Not attributed to another disorder

headache of a nonmigrainous nature. Less treatable mimics of NDPH include posttraumatic headache (see Chapter 28) and postmeningitis headache.

Diagnostic investigation in this patient should therefore probably include magnetic resonance imaging of the brain before and after gadolinium, lumbar puncture with measurement of opening pressure and CSF analysis for infectious or inflammatory causes, and systemic screening for infectious and inflammatory disease including erythrocyte sedimentation rate, Lyme titer, lupus testing, VDRL, complete blood count, and serum chemistry screening. Thyroid screening, as well as screening for diabetes, is sensible if there are suggestive features. (This patient was tachycardic—perhaps related to a hyperthyroid state.)

As for the etiology of the primary form of NDPH, this is entirely unclear. The fact that many cases can be traced to a viral illness suggests that an infectious process may have altered head nociceptive physiology in some way (similar to a suggested etiology for the fibromyalgia syndrome). Or perhaps, as Evans and Rosen (2001) have suggested, the initial viral infection may have altered the immune system to promote a persistent inflammatory state. A significant fraction of patients with NDPH have Epstein-Barr viral antibodies, denoting previous infection. But a previous or preceding viral infection might simply be coincidental. Might there have been mild head trauma in some cases that patients discounted? In the case above, perhaps having "slept badly" was indicative of some cervical structural problem. Rozen and Swiden (2007) found recently that CSF tumor necrosis factor-α (TNF-α) levels were increased in all of a group of NDPH patients, suggestive of central nervous system inflammation. (Interestingly, TNF-α levels were also increased in their control group consisting of chronic migraine and posttraumatic headache patients). Or could NDPH simply represent a subtype of chronic migraine or chronic tension-type headache with more abrupt onset than usual? These issues will hopefully be sorted out as reliable biochemical, imaging, and other markers for the primary headaches emerge.

Treatment in NDPH is generally never fully effective (another good reason to search for a treatable cause). Virtually all migraine prophylactic agents have been tried, with varying results, including tricyclic antidepressants, selective serotonin reuptake inhibitors, beta-blockers, calcium channel blockers, antiepileptic drugs (particularly gabapentin, topiramate, and valproate), antispasmodics, and muscle relaxants. Intravenous dihydroergotamine has been proposed as a several-day course to interrupt the cycle of daily headaches and has been successful in some cases. This could be of use in the patient here, along with the institution of a novel prophylactic agent, perhaps in the anticonvulsant category. Botulinum toxin has been tried anecdotally in a number of cases of NDPH, with mixed results.

Medication overuse is frequently a real problem, for obvious reasons, and must be dealt with in order to have a chance at successful outcome.

With patients like the one summarized above, it is important to stress the importance of nonpharmacological pain-reducing techniques like relaxation training and lifestyle adjustment (sleep regulation, regular exercise, etc.) and to remain optimistic about continuing the search for the best prophylactic program, which may include polypharmacy. Counseling can be important when patients become demoralized. Procedures like occipital nerve blocks and even transcranial magnetic stimulation may have promise but remain unproven. Some cases do remit on their own.

KEY POINTS TO REMEMBER

- New daily persistent headache resembles chronic tension-type headache, with few migraine features but an identifiable time of onset.
- A number of occult mimics must be ruled out in these cases despite the benign appearance of most patients.
- There may be two clinical subtypes: a self-limited form and a refractory persistent form.
- Treatment is unsatisfactory in most patients, although some degree of pain reduction is almost always achievable.

Further Reading

Evans RW, Rosen TD. Etiology and treatment of new daily persistent headache. Headache 2001;41:830–832.

Rozen T, Swiden SZ. Elevation of CSF tumor necrosis factor levels in new daily persistent headache and treatment refractory chronic migraine. Headache 2007;47:1050–1055.

Rozen TD. Successful treatment of new daily-persistent headache with gabapentin and topiramate. Headache 2002;42:433.

Takase Y, Nakano M, Tatsumi C, Matsuyama T. Clinical features, effectiveness of drug-based treatment, and prognosis of new daily persistent headache (NDPH): 30 cases in Japan. Cephalalgia 2004;24(11):955–959.

Vanast WJ. New daily-persistent headaches: definition of a benign syndrome. Headache 1986;26:318.

Spontaneous Intracranial Hypotension

A 48-year-old woman presents with a new-onset headache that began after weeding in her garden. These headaches are global and throbbing, of moderate severity, and associated with neck pain and stiffness. The headaches are strictly positional in that they worsen with standing and resolve when she lays down. Her exam is entirely normal. A lumbar puncture, done in the sitting position, reveals an opening pressure of 40 mm H_2O. Contrast-enhanced magnetic resonance imaging (MRI) of the brain reveals pachymeningeal enhancement (Fig. 9-1). Treatment with non-steroidal anti-inflammatory drugs, intravenous caffeine, and multiple blood patches failed to relieve the pain.

What do you do now?

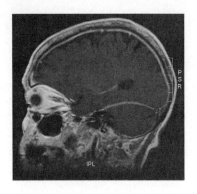

FIGURE 9-1 Pachymeningeal enhancement. (Courtesy of Gordon Heller, MD, Department of Neuro-Radiology, Roosevelt Hospital Center, New York, NY)

Spontaneous intracranial hypotension (SIH) is a well-recognized syndrome that is characterized by orthostatic headaches in association with a variety of other symptoms. The syndrome is caused by an occult leakage of cerebrospinal fluid (CSF), which produces a decrease in CSF volume and subsequently intracranial hypotension. Unlike the low-CSF pressure syndromes that result from lumbar punctures or dural fistulas, SIH by definition begins without an identifiable precipitant. This disorder should be included in the differential diagnosis of any patient who complains of new onset of daily persistent headaches, as well as patients with refractory daily headache, especially if there is a positional element.

The characteristic clinical feature of SIH is headache. The typical headache is positional in that the pain worsens with sitting or standing and lessens with recumbency. The longer the patient remains upright, the longer it takes for the headache to dissipate when lying down. The headaches are usually throbbing, bilateral, and worsened by Valsalva maneuvers. Although this orthostatic headache is classic for this syndrome, other nonorthostatic presentations are possible. Also, a previously orthostatic headache may become chronic and unremitting over time, losing the positionality. The headaches may be associated with neck stiffness, tinnitus, hypacusia, photophobia, intrascapular pain, nausea, vomiting, blurred vision, and diplopia (secondary to cranial nerve palsies).

The incidence of SIH is not known; it may be underrecognized by many clinicians, especially when the patient presents with long-standing symptoms. Often, the diagnosis is made accidentally when a patient with daily headaches is found to have features of SIH on the MRI. In the majority of cases, the cause of SIH is unclear, but possible precipitants include a history of trivial trauma and weakness of the dural sac. The traumatic event is typically minor and includes coughing, straining, sexual activity, lifting, bending, minor falls, sports injuries, and gardening. The dural sac weakness may be the result of connective tissue disorders (Marfan, Ehlers-Danlos syndromes) or meningeal diverticula; in fact, 16%–38% of patients with SIH are noted to have connective tissue disorders.

Leaks of CSF in SIH are usually found in the thoracic spine but at times are seen at the cervical or lumbar levels. These leaks frequently occur along the dural root sleeves, and meningeal diverticula are often noted at these levels as well. In some patients, the leaks occur intracranially rather than in the spinal cord. The leakage of CSF results in a decrease in the total CSF volume, which causes sinking of the brain in the skull. This "brain sag" induces traction on the pain-sensitive suspending and anchoring structures of the brain and is responsible for the headache and associated signs and symptoms of this disorder. The positional component of the headache is the result of the increase in the downward displacement of the brain and the increase in traction upon the pain-sensitive structures that occurs in a gravity-dependent manner when the patient assumes an upright position. Traction upon cranial nerves III–VIII and the brainstem results in nerve palsies and mental status changes, whereas the changes in pressure that are transmitted into the perilymphatic fluid produce the tinnitus, hypacusia, and vestibular complaints.

The diagnosis of SIH may be established in a number of ways. Brain MRI without gadolinium may demonstrate "brain sag," descent of the cerebellar tonsils (pseudo-Chiari I), a decrease in the prepontine or perichiasmatic cisterns, flattening of the optic chiasm, posterior fossa crowding, a decrease in the size of the ventricles, subdural collections, and enlargement of the venous sinuses. Contrast-enhanced MRI typically shows diffuse pachymeningeal, but not leptomeningeal, enhancement. Pachymeningeal enhancement is not always present and may disappear over time; therefore, it is not required for the diagnosis. Spine MRI may demonstrate extra-arachnoid fluid collections, meningeal diverticula, pachymeningeal enhancement (usually cervical), and engorgement of the spinal epidural venous plexus. Radioisotope cisternography using indium 111 may demonstrate the site of the CSF leak. Abnormal findings include early uptake of the radioisotope in the kidneys or bladder as the result of extravasation from the subarachnoid space into the paraspinal soft tissues and failure or delay of the isotope to reach the cerebral convexities. Normally, the isotope will reach the convexities within 24 hours, but in the presence of a leak it may be delayed up to 48 hours or longer. Computed tomographic (CT) myelography can also demonstrate the site of the CSF leak as evidenced by extradural contrast extravasation, meningeal diverticula, or extra-arachnoid collections of CSF. According to the *International Classification of Headache Disorders*, second edition criteria, lumbar puncture should be done with the patient in a seated position. To do this properly, the patient is placed in a seated position with neck and spine maximally flexed and arms resting on a bedside table. Drawing an imaginary line between the two posterior iliac crests will approximate the L4–L5 or L3–L4 interspace. When measuring the opening pressure, a water manometer is attached to the spinal needle via a three-way stopcock. Unlike the normal pressures measured with the patient in the lateral decubitus position (65–195 mm H_2O), in the seated position the normal pressure is approximately 280 mm H_2O. The opening pressure in patients with SIH is usually very low ($\leq$60 mm H_2O) or unmeasurable. In 40% of patients with SIH, the pressures are consistently within the normal range. The CSF is usually normal but may show elevated protein, white blood cell, or red blood cell counts. In general, lumbar puncture is not performed early in the work-up of SIH because it may worsen the clinical picture and because removing fluid may cause pachymeningeal enhancement on MRI.

Treatment of SIH includes conservative measures such as bed rest and hydration and caffeine administration (by mouth or intravenously). Epidural blood patching, in which the patient is injected with 10–20 cc of autologous blood in the lumbar epidural region, may provide relief. Some patients require repeated blood patches for relief. Success rates for the first patch range 30%–56%, and the efficacy of each subsequent patch is approximately 30%. About half of the patients who do not respond to the first or second patch will respond to additional patches. Success rates are enhanced if the patches are targeted to the site of leakage that was demonstrated on cisternography or myelography. If repeated blood patches are unsuccessful and the site of the leak is known, percutaneous placement of 4–20 ml of fibrin sealant injected via a transforaminal approach may offer relief. For refractory cases, surgical exploration and repair is necessary.

Our patient has clinical features and diagnostic studies that indicate SIH. As she has failed conservative methods and repeated blood patches, further testing to identify the site of the leak is needed. If a leak site is identified, then targeted blood patching should be tried, followed by percutaneous fibrin injections. If these are unhelpful, then surgical exploration and repair should be attempted. Although our patient most likely has a spinal localization of her leak, some patients have an intracranial leak. These patients may complain of rhinorrhea, although in some patients the CSF is inadvertently swallowed. If CSF rhinorrhea is present, the use of nasal pledgets should be included in the radionuclide cisternography searching for radioactivity. The nasal secretions should also be collected and tested for glucose and beta-2 transferrin. In these patients, the CSF leak may be identified through thin-cut CT scans, nasal endoscopy, or cisternography and surgical correction can be curative.

KEY POINTS TO REMEMBER

- Spontaneous intracranial hypotension results from an occult leak of CSF usually without precipitant.
- Spontaneous intracranial hypotension may be preceded by trivial trauma.
- Some patients have a connective tissue disorder.
- Opening pressure is usually below 60 mm H_2O in the sitting position, but 40% of patients have normal opening pressure.
- Contrast-enhanced MRI demonstrates enhancement of the pachymeninges but not the leptomeninges.
- Site of leak may be seen with indium 111 cisternography or CT myelography.
- Blood patching success rates are 30%–56% for the first patch but 30% for each subsequent patch, so subsequent trials should be attempted if the first fails.

Further Reading

Mokri B. Low CSF pressure syndromes. Neurol Clin North Am 2004;22:55-74.

Mokri B. Spontaneous low cerebrospinal pressure/volume headaches. Curr Neurol Neurosci Rep 2004;4:117-124.

Schievink WI, Maya MM, Moser FM. Treatment of spontaneous intracranial hypotension with percutaneous placement of a fibrin sealant: report of four cases. J Neurosurg 2004;100:1098-1100.

Schwedt TJ, Dodick DW. Spontaneous intracranial hypotension. Curr Pain Headache Rep 2007;11:56-61.

10 Vasculitis Headache

A 31-year-old man began to experience headaches in various areas of the head 3 months ago. Headaches can occur suddenly, and on several occasions he has had transient weakness or sensory loss in a limb but does not recall locations. The location of the headache tends to be posterior but varies. He denies nausea, vomiting, photophobia, and phonophobia. Neurological exam is entirely normal other than for some anxiety. Head magnetic resonance imaging (MRI) and lumbar puncture after a particularly severe headache were negative. Triptans have been of minimal help.

What do you do now?

This case is worrisome for several reasons. First, this is a new headache in a patient who has not had headaches in the past—although not unheard of, and certainly age 31 is a possible time for onset of a number of primary headaches. Second, there are symptoms of neurological compromise in nonstereotypical locations (See Table 10–1 for clues which suggest possible intracranial pathology). Transient neurological symptoms are clues to one of four categories in neurological disease: (1) cerebral ischemic disease, (2) epilepsy (partial seizures), (3) migraine, and on occasion (4) mass lesions. It is not clear how mass lesions cause symptoms which come and go, but perhaps vascular or metabolic phenomena are involved. The normal MRI here essentially excludes mass lesions. Recurrent intracerebral hemorrhages or subarachnoid bleeding is probably also ruled out by the normal MRI and clear cerebrospinal fluid (CSF). However there is the specter of symptomatic unruptured aneurysms or aneurysmal "sentinel" bleeding, both of which may have been missed. Partial seizures with "negative" phenomena (numbness and weakness, as opposed to tonic or clonic movements) are unusual but not impossible, and electroencephalography might be worth considering, particularly during an episode. Migraine without nausea and phono-/photophobia is distinctly unlikely, and true weakness as an aura symptom (hemiplegic migraine) is quite rare.

Cerebrovascular disease is not uncommonly associated with headache. This patient is young for the usual causes of transient ischemic attack or

TABLE 10-1   **Red Flags in the Presentation of Headache (That Warrant Further Investigation)**

- New onset
- Change in pattern of preexisting headaches
- Effort induced
- Positional
- Onset in middle age or later
- Febrile
- Change in behavior or cognition
- Neurological symptoms unusual for migraine aura
- Neurological findings
- Setting of systemic illness (e.g., AIDS, cancer)

stroke, but hyperviscosity, hypercoagulability, cardiac sources of embolism, and inflammatory causes of cerebral ischemia should be ruled out. Serological work-up of possible coagulation defects as well as echocardiography and MRI of the cervical vessels seems sensible. Vasculitis of the central nervous system (CNS), whether localized to the head or part of a systemic condition, typically causes headache along with neurological deficits; but CSF is almost always remarkable for cellularity and increased protein. Still, vasculitis can be occult; and causes include infectious (HIV, herpes zoster, or fungal, parasitic, or treponemal meningitis), drugs, lymphoma, Behçet disease, polyarteritis nodosa, Churg-Strauss disease, and Wegener granulomatosis (see Table 10–2). Cerebral venous thrombosis is another possible cause of transient neurological deficits and sudden headaches, often missed on standard MRI, so MR venography would be sensible in cases such as this one.

This patient's syndrome is, in fact, most typical of the so-called reversible cerebral vasoconstriction syndromes (RCVS). These represent a group of disorders characterized by recurring acute headaches and reversible vasoconstriction of cerebral arteries, leading to neurological signs and symptoms of various degrees, presenting over days to weeks. There are a number of synonyms for the general syndrome including Call–Fleming syndrome, benign angiopathy of the CNS, and thunderclap headache

TABLE 10-2   **Vasculitis Affecting the Cerebral Vessels**

A. Cerebral vasculitis
    1. Primary angiitis of the central nervous system
    2. HIV, herpes zoster
    3. Meningitic–fungal, parasitic, or treponemal
    4. Drug-induced–amphetamines, cocaine
    5. Lymphoma
    6. Giant cell arteritis–extradural arteries only

B. Systemic vasculitis which may affect cerebral arteries
    1. Behçet–often with genital/oral ulcers, arthritis, ocular signs
    2. Polyarteritis nodosa–often with fever, arthralgias, myalgias, mononeuropathies
    3. Churg-Strauss–often with asthma, eosinophilia, neuropathy
    4. Wegener–often with neuropathy
    5. Systemic lupus erythematosus–generally with fever, rash, arthritis, pleuritis, encephalopathy

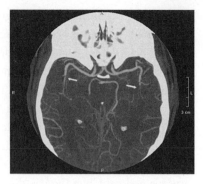

FIGURE 10-1 Cerebral angiogram showing the typical segmental arterial narrowing seen in reversible cerebral vasoconstriction syndrome (RCVS). (Courtesy of David W. Dodick, MD, Department of Neurology, Mayo Clinic, Scottsdale, AZ.)

with reversible vasospasm. Probably, RCVS includes a number of cases of drug-induced cerebral arteritis. The etiology of RCVS is not clear, but it can occur coincidently with certain medication or drug use or in pregnancy. It is differentiated from primary angiitis of the CNS by its normal CSF. It is diagnosed by reversible segmental cerebral arterial constriction on angiography. One other candidate for this patient's diagnosis is the mysterious condition: headache with associated neurological deficits and CSF lymphocytosis (HaNDL). Like RCVS, patients with HaNDL have transient neurological deficits, but they generally have more typical migraine headaches (hence the synonym "pseudomigraine"), increased CSF protein and pressure, and CSF pleocytosis (lymphocytic). Patients with HaNDL have no prior history of migraine, and their condition is generally self-limited (maximum of 3 months). Recent evidence seems to link HaNDL to migraine pathophysiology.

In this patient, repeat lumbar puncture is a reasonable idea to see if CSF protein is high or if there is a pleocytosis. Angiography should be done, and the decision about standard direct angiography versus computed tomography (CT) or MR angiography will have to be made. Probably, high-quality CT angiography is sufficient to rule out the segmental arterial narrowing of RCVS or cerebral arteritis (see Fig. 10–1).

If RCVS is diagnosed, indicated treatment is thought to include the calcium channel blockers nimodipine or verapamil and possibly corticosteroids. Interestingly, with support, most patients do very well with minimal presistence of neurological deficits.

- With generally healthy individuals and a normal neurological examination, most headache presentations are benign.
- "Red flags" warrant further neurological work-up, including imaging, vascular, and CSF studies.
- Central nervous system vasculitis virtually always includes headache of some type.
- Generally, RCVS, a mimic of CNS vasculitis, is self-limited and CSF is normal.

Further Reading

Calabrese LH, Dodick DW, Schwedt TJ, Singhal AB. Narrative review. Reversible cerebral vasoconstriction syndromes. Ann Intern Med 2007;146:34-44.

Edmeads J. Headache related to cerebrovascular disease. In: Levin M, Ward TN (eds), Head, Neck and Facial Pain. Columbus, OH: Anadem, 2006.

Fumal A, Vandenheede M, Coppola G, et al. The syndrome of transient headache with neurological deficits and CSF lymphocytosis (HaNDL): electrophysiological findings suggestive of migrainous pathophysiology. Cephalalgia 2005;25:754-758.

Lie JT. Classification and histopathologic spectrum of central nervous system vasculitis. Neurol Clin 1997;15(4):805-819.

Migraine with Persistent Aura

A 40-year-old man with a history of migraine with visual aura since his teens reports that several weeks ago he developed his typical headache that was preceded by scintillating scotoma in his left visual field. That aura, like all his others, lasted 30 minutes and was followed by a hemicranial, throbbing headache. The migraine headache resolved within 1 hour of treatment with rizatriptan; however, the aura recurred soon after and has been fluctuating in size but never completely disappearing. The headache has not recurred, and no other neurological complaints are reported. He has no prior medical history and is on no other medication. Computed tomography of the head is normal. An ophthalmological evaluation was normal, as was an electroencephalography. The patient is quite disabled by the visual phenomena and has been afraid to drive his car for the past 3 weeks. He fears that he has had a stroke.

What do you do now?

Approximately 20% of migraine sufferers experience an aura with their headaches. Auras are characterized by transient episodes of fully reversible focal neurological disturbances that may precede or accompany the headache. Occasionally, auras may occur without headache. In general, auras develop gradually over 5–20 minutes and resolve within an hour or less. The migraine aura may manifest as a visual, sensory, or language disturbance and may be simple or complex (Table 11–1). The *International Classification of Headache Disorders*, second edition (ICHD-II), classification of migraine with aura (Table 11–2) excludes motor disturbances as an aura phenomenon; when motor weakness occurs as part of an aura, the diagnosis of familial or sporadic hemiplegic migraine should be considered.

Most auras are of a visual nature and may present as photopsias or *phosphenes* (unformed flashes of lights), geometric forms, shimmering waves, or scotoma (positive or negative). Visual auras are usually bilateral and slowly move across the visual field. The classic visual aura, the fortification spectrum, is characterized by a zigzag or herringbone pattern at the point of visual fixation. Over time, this shape enlarges to encroach upon the visual hemifield, assuming a jagged, convex shape. The borders of the spectrum

TABLE 11-1 **Migraine Auras**

Visual
Photopsias
Phosphenes
Scotomata
Geometric shapes
Fortification spectra
Micro-/macropsia
Mosaic vision
Metamorphopsia
Sensory
Paresthesias
Cheiro-oral numbness
Olfactory/gustatory/auditory hallucinations
Speech
Dysphasic
Dysarthric
Aphasic

TABLE 11-2 **Typical Aura with Migraine Headache**

Description

Typical aura consisting of visual and/or sensory and/or speech symptoms. Gradual development, duration no longer than 1 hour, a mix of positive and negative features, and complete reversibility characterize the aura which is associated with a headache fulfilling criteria for migraine without aura.

Diagnostic criteria

A. At least two attacks fulfilling criteria B–D

B. Aura consisting of at least one of the following but no motor weakness:
1. Fully reversible visual symptoms including positive features (e.g., flickering lights, spots, or lines) and/or negative features (i.e., loss of vision)
2. Fully reversible sensory symptoms including positive features (i.e., pins and needles) and/or negative features (i.e., numbness)
3. Fully reversible dysphasic speech disturbance

C. At least two of the following:
1. Homonymous visual symptoms[1] and/or unilateral sensory symptoms
2. At least one aura symptom develops gradually over ≥5 minutes and/or different aura symptoms occur in succession over ≥5 minutes
3. Each symptom lasts ≥5 and ≤60 minutes

D. Headache fulfilling criteria B–D for migraine without aura begins during the aura or follows aura within 60 minutes

E. Not attributed to another disorder[2]

---

[1] Additional loss or blurring of central vision may occur.

[2] History and physical and neurological examinations do not suggest any of the disorders listed in groups 5–12; or history and/or physical and/or neurological examinations do suggest such disorder, but it is ruled out by appropriate investigations or is present but attacks do not occur for the first time in close temporal relation to the disorder.

---

typically are shimmering, composed of flashing lights, jagged lines, or geometric patterns that surround a blind spot (*scotoma*) that may occupy the center of the design. *Metamorphopsia* is an abnormality in visual perception in which the shapes or borders of objects become distorted or disjointed. Patients who have metamorphoptic auras often report that objects appear smaller (*micropsia*) or larger (*macropsia*) than they really are. These patients may note that objects appear to be farther away (*telopsia*). Other common auras include sensory disturbances (paresthesias, numbness). The typical sensory aura, cheiro-oral numbness, is characterized by paresthesias that begin in the hand, slowly march upward to involve the forearm, and then produce numbness of the ipsilateral face, lip, and chin. Language disturbances usually manifest as dysphasic speech; true aphasia is very rare.

Rarely, the migraine aura may persist for extended periods of time. The ICHD-II now designates two subclasses of prolonged aura. When one or more aura symptoms continue for more than an hour and there is evidence of an ischemic lesion in the appropriate site on neuroimaging, the diagnosis of migrainous infarction is used. If the aura symptoms persist for more than 1 week without radiographic evidence of a stroke, then the diagnosis is persistent aura without infarction. Patients suffering from very prolonged auras, in which aura symptoms recur repeatedly on a daily basis or persist unabated for months or years, have been described and are often referred to as being in "migraine aura status."

Obviously, any patient who suffers from a prolonged neurological deficit requires a complete work-up including neuroimaging, to rule out cerebrovascular disease. Other disorders which may mimic prolonged auras include occipital lobe epilepsy; vertebrobasilar transient ischemic attacks; posterior leukoencephalopathy; carotid or vertebral artery dissection (see Chapter 6); retinal detachment; hematological diseases (polycythemia vera); hyperhomocysteinemia; mitochondrial encephalopathy, lactic acidosis, and stroke-like episodes (MELAS) syndrome; and cerebral autosomal dominant arteriopathy with subcortical infarcts and leukoencephalopathy (CADASIL).

Our patient has had a continuous visual aura for the past 3 weeks. Although his neurological examination is normal, we must order magnetic resonance imaging (MRI) of the brain, to rule out secondary mimics such as infarction or posterior leukoencephalopathy, and blood work, to screen for blood dyscrasias, increased homocysteine levels, and autoimmune disorders. Since his visual disturbances are apparently in both eyes, dissection is unlikely. A normal MRI would essentially rule out CADASIL. This patient seems to meet the criteria for persistent aura without infarction.

There is no standard treatment protocol for patients suffering from prolonged auras (Table 11–3). Older therapies reported to demonstrate success in individual patients include inhalation therapy with 10% carbon dioxide and 90% oxygen, amyl nitrate or isoproterenol, and sublingual nifedipine. These treatments were based on the theory that migrainous auras were the result of prolonged vasoconstriction. Aura is now believed to be the result of cortical spreading depression, and treatments aimed at interfering with

TABLE 11-3   **Treatment of Prolonged Auras**

Older therapies
Inhalation of 10% CO_2 and 90% O_2
Inhalation of amyl nitrate
Inhalation of isoproterenol
Sublingual nifedipine 10 mg

Newer therapies (based on cortical spreading depression model)
IV furosemide 20 mg
Oral acetazolamide 500-750 mg daily
Intranasal ketamine 25 mg
IV prochlorperazine 10 mg q 8 hours with magnesium sulfate 1 g q 12 hours

Source: Rozen 2003

this mechanism include intravenous furosemide, magnesium sulfate and prochlorperazine, and intranasal ketamine. Oral divalproex, acetazolamide, verapamil, flunarizine, lamotrigine, gabapentin, and memantine have also been reported to be beneficial.

KEY POINTS TO REMEMBER

- Migrainous aura occurs in approximately 20% of migraine sufferers and is usually a visual, sensory, or language disturbance.
- Motor auras are not typical of migraine.
- Migrainous aura develop over 5-20 minutes and resolve within 1 hour or less.
- Rarely, auras persist for extended periods of time; these are divided as follows:
  - *Migrainous infarction:* When one or more aura symptoms continue for more than an hour and there is evidence of an ischemic lesion in the appropriate site on neuroimaging.
  - *Persistent aura without infarction*: Aura symptoms persisting for more than 1 week without radiographic evidence of a stroke.

Further Reading
Agostini E, Aliprandi A. Complications of migraine with aura. Neurol. Sci. 2006;27:S91-S95.
Haas DC. Prolonged migraine aura status. Ann. Neurol. 1982;11:197-199.
Rozen TD. Aborting a prolonged migrainous aura with intravenous prochlorperazine and magnesium sulfate. Headache 2003;43:901-903.

Migrainous Vertigo

A 47-year-old man describes bouts of severe vertigo during which he is completely disabled. He has had episodes as brief as 5 minutes and as long as 4–5 hours. There is often nausea, but he usually does not vomit. He has had diarrhea as an accompaniment on a few occasions and has also had bitemporal headaches with a few of these spells. He denies any other symptoms, such as motor, sensory, visual, or balance dysfunction. He has failed to respond to meclizine, and an otolaryngologist has decided this is "migrainous vertigo" (MV). Magnetic resonance imaging (MRI) is normal, and both electroencephalography (EEG) and audiometry are likewise normal. The one thing that has helped him is intravenous chlorpromazine, which was used in an emergency room once. His examination is normal.

What do you do now?

Vertigo and migraine have a number of associations. Vertigo is a relatively common, although generally mild, aura symptom in patients with migraine with aura. A childhood syndrome felt to be closely related to migraine, benign paroxysmal vertigo of childhood, occurs in the absence of headache, although a family history of migraine is common and these children are very likely to develop migraine. (This syndrome is characterized by recurrent brief bouts of vertigo and nausea, with intervening asymptomatic periods.) Many patients with migraine suffer from motion sickness, including the merely visually induced variety (e.g., watching widescreen movies). Finally, basilar-type migraine (BTM) is commonly accompanied by vertigo. This type of migraine (which has never actually been shown to be due to any change in the basilar artery) is diagnosed by very specific criteria (Table 12–1). First, migraine headaches have to occur along with several aura symptoms, including dysarthria, vertigo, tinnitus, reduced hearing (*hypacusia*), diplopia, bilateral visual field manifestations, ataxia, decreased consciousness, and bilateral limb/trunk sensation changes.

TABLE 12-1   ICHD II Diagnostic Criteria for Basilar-Type Migraine 1.2.6

A. At least two attacks fulfilling criteria B-D

B. Aura consisting of at least two of the following fully reversible symptoms but no motor weakness:
   1. Dysarthria
   2. Vertigo
   3. Tinnitus
   4. Hypacusia
   5. Diplopia
   6. Visual symptoms simultaneously in both temporal and nasal fields of both eyes
   7. Ataxia
   8. Decreased level of consciousness
   9. Simultaneous bilateral paraesthesias

C. At least one of the following:
   1. At least one aura symptom develops gradually over ≥5 minutes and/or different aura symptoms occur in succession over ≥5 minutes
   2. Each aura symptom lasts ≥5 and ≤60 minutes

D. Headache fulfilling criteria B-D for migraine without aura begins during the aura or follows aura within 60 minutes

E. Not attributed to another disorder

Recurrent vertigo without headache as a migraine form in adults is controversial but has long been discussed in the literature. There are no known biological or clinical markers, but proposed definitions of MV generally include the following:

1. Recurrent bouts of vertigo lasting minutes to hours
2. Current or past diagnosis of migraine
3. Several migraine headaches or migraine symptoms, like photophobia, phonophobia, or other aura symptoms, occurring in close proximity to the vertigo spells

How might migraine produce vertigo? This is not known, but a number of clever explanations have been proposed: (*1*) cortical spreading depression in the region of the lateral temporal lobe (known to be a site where other pathological processes can produce vertigo), (*2*) migraine-induced reduction of regional blood flow involving the circulation of the inner ear, and (*3*) release of vasoactive peptides by trigeminal nerve endings in the vicinity of the inner ear, resulting in changes in vestibular neural activity.

In evaluating patients with possible MV the first step is to decide if the symptoms do indeed represent true vertigo rather than light-headedness, ataxia, or panic. This is generally not too challenging if the differences are explained to patients. Illnesses which present with episodic vertigo that can mimic MV include Meniere disease, benign positional vertigo (BPV), BTM (as mentioned above), perilymphatic fistula, demyelinating disease (with plaque[s] in the region of vestibular nuclei), transient ischemic attacks, and acoustic nerve region tumors (schwannoma, meningioma, epidermoid) (Table 12–2). Meniere disease involves some degree of hearing loss, as is commonly true for acoustic nerve masses, which is much less likely in migraine. Unlike MV, BPV is produced by position change (e.g., with Hallpike maneuver). Acute labyrinthitis, or vestibular neuronitis, is a single episode and is longer-lasting than MV. In short, when other causes of recurrent vertigo seem unlikely, it is worth considering MV and treating as such . Finally, it is important to remember that since migraine is much more common in Meniere disease and BPV than in the general population, patients like the one in the case above could simply have a combination of migraine and either of these.

TABLE 12-2 Differential Diagnosis of Recurrent Vertigo (with Diagnostic Clues)

Condition	Clues to Diagnosis
Basilar migraine	Concurrent migraine headache and other aura symptoms reflecting posterior circulation regions
Benign positional vertigo	Strictly brought on by head position change
Vestibular neuronitis/labyrinthitis	Single episode, hours to days
Meniere disease	Hearing loss and/or tinnitus
Posttraumatic vertigo	History of trauma, symptoms similar to benign positional vertigo
Phobic/psychogenic vertigo	Situational, history of anxiety, no nystagmus
Perilymphatic fistula	History of antecedent barotrauma, forceful nose blowing, sneeze, etc.; hearing loss
Labyrinthine or brainstem ischemia	Other signs of neurological dysfunction
Meningitis–carcinomatous, tuberculous, fungal	Other cranial nerve dysfunction, meningismus
Brainstem or cerebellopontine tumor	Hearing loss, signs of brainstem dysfunction
Complex partial seizures	History of epilepsy, abnormal electroencephalogram
Vertebrobasilar ischemia	Signs of brainstem dysfunction such as facial numbness, diplopia, dysarthria, Horner syndrome
Multiple sclerosis–brainstem plaque	Other neurological signs and symptoms
Medication effect–aspirin, phenytoin, aminoglycosides, cisplatin	Correlates with medication changes, constant
Migrainous vertigo	History of migraine, aura, or other migraine symptoms; accompanied by headache

The patient above seems to have MV. There are no accompanying neurological deficits, there are headaches associated with some spells, and the time course is right. Basic evaluation has already included negative MRI, audiometry, and EEG. Careful Hallpike maneuver testing should be done. It is worth remembering that many patients with migraine with aura find their headaches becoming rarer as they get older but that auras continue to occur. This patient is the right age for this phenomenon and may have had migraines in the past. (A good question to ask.)

Treatment of MV can be very gratifying. Elimination of triggers (e.g., sleep deprivation, ingested substances) is very important and may serve as the key therapeutic approach. Acute attacks may respond to meclizine or dimenhydrinate (Dramamine), but these are usually not sufficient. Promethazine and metoclopramide are better in general. Triptans have been useful for many patients when taken soon after the vertigo begins, which stands to reason, although there is no evidence yet to support their use. For prophylaxis, betablockers, calcium channel blockers, tricyclic antidepressants, clonazepam, topiramate, and lamotrigine have been successful in selected cases. We have personally found nortriptyline 25–50 mg qhs, topiramate 50–200 mg daily in two divided doses, and a combination of amitriptyline and chlordiazepoxide (Limbitrol) 12.5mg/5 mg qhs to be useful.

KEY POINTS TO REMEMBER

- Migrainous vertigo should be considered in patients in whom other causes of recurrent vertigo have been excluded or are unlikely.
- Generally, patients have a clear history of migraine and at least several occasions when both migraine headache and vertigo co-occurred.
- Treatment for MV is similar to that for migraine headache— elimination of triggers, acute treatment, and prophylactic medication.

Further Reading

Eggers SDZ. Migraine-related vertigo: diagnosis and treatment. Curr Pain Headache Rep 2007;11:217-226.

Johnson GD. Medical management of migraine-related dizziness and vertigo. Laryngoscope 1998;108(suppl 85):1-28.

Neuhauser H, Leopold M, von Brevern M. The interrelations of migraine, vertigo, and migrainous vertigo. Neurology 2001;56:436-441.

Vucovic V, Plavec D, Galinovic L, et al. Prevalence of vertigo, dizziness, and migrainous vertigo in patients with migraine. Headache 2007;47:1427-1435.

13 Cough Headache

A 48-year-old man presents with a 2-week history of
headache that developed during an upper respiratory
illness. The headaches come on abruptly whenever he
coughs or sneezes and are characterized by a sharp,
stabbing sensation at the vertex and occiput lasting
from 20 seconds to 2 minutes. At times, a dull headache
lingers for several hours afterward. He denies nausea,
vomiting, photophobia, or phonophobia and has no
prior or family history of headaches. At times, these
headaches may be triggered by lifting heavy packages.
He is exhausted, having been awakened multiple times
nightly by coughing fits and headaches. His medical
exam is remarkable only for scattered rhonchi. The
neurological examination is entirely normal.

What do you do now?

This case is a cause for concern in that the headaches are of new onset and begin for the first time in a middle-aged man. Additionally, these headaches occur suddenly and follow maneuvers that increase intracranial pressure. Although the neurological examination is normal, the clinical history is suspicious for an intracranial lesion (see "Red Flags," Chapter 24).

Headaches that occur with coughing, sneezing, straining, or exertion should prompt a search for lesions within the posterior fossa, craniocervical junction, or cerebrospinal fluid (CSF) pathways. Although cough and exertional headaches are often linked together as "Valsalva maneuver headaches," they are distinct entities within the *International Classification of Headache Disorders*, second edition (ICHD-II), classification. The diagnosis of the primary forms of these disorders can only be made after secondary forms have been excluded. Hence, neuroimaging is required.

Primary cough headache is uncommon, with a lifetime prevalence of approximately 1%. This condition typically affects men over 40 years of age, and while often described as a severe headache of sudden onset, it is by definition benign. Within seconds of coughing, sneezing, straining, or other Valsalva maneuvers, an immediate headache is experienced. The headache usually subsides within 1 second to 30 minutes; however, some sufferers may continue to experience a dull ache for several hours afterward. The pain is usually described as sharp, stabbing, or splitting in nature; of moderate to severe intensity; and generally bilateral. The pain is usually reported to be maximally felt at the vertex, frontal, occipital, or temporal areas and is unassociated with neurological symptoms, nausea, or vomiting. The ICHD-II diagnostic criteria for primary cough headache are listed in Table 13–1. While the precise etiology is unknown, it may relate to a sudden increase in intracranial pressure with traction on pain-sensitive structures from a downward displacement of cerebellar tonsils.

When cough headache occurs in a younger patient, is of long duration, is strictly unilateral, or is associated with other features, the diagnosis must be questioned. Secondary cough headache has been described in Chiari malformation (Chapter 7); brain tumors, both malignant and benign (meningioma/ acoustic neuroma); cerebral aneurysm; and carotid or vertebrobasilar disease.

Primary exertional headache, not surprisingly, occurs with exertional effort, as may occur during physical exercise, weight lifting, straining, or bending over. The headache is of sudden onset and often bilateral in

TABLE 13-1   **Primary Cough Headache**

Previously used terms

Benign cough headache, Valsalva-maneuver headache

Description

Headache precipitated by coughing or straining in the absence of any intracranial disorder

Diagnostic criteria

A. Headache fulfilling criteria B and C

B. Sudden onset, lasting 1 second to 30 minutes

C. Brought on by and occurring only in association with coughing, straining, and/or Valsalva maneuver

D. Not attributed to another disorder[1]

[1] Is symptomatic in about 40% of cases, and the large majority of these present Arnold-Chiari malformation type I. Other reported causes of symptomatic cough headache include carotid or vertebrobasilar diseases and cerebral aneurysms. Diagnostic neuroimaging plays an important role in differentiating secondary cough headache from primary cough headache.

TABLE 13-2   **Primary Exertional Headache**

Description

Headache precipitated by any form of exercise

Diagnostic criteria

A. Pulsating headache fulfilling criteria B and C

B. Lasting 5 minutes to 48 hours

C. Brought on by and occurring only during or after physical exertion

D. Not attributed to another disorder[1]

[1] On first occurrence of this headache type, it is mandatory to exclude subarachnoid hemorrhage and arterial dissection.

location, but unlike cough headache, the pain is often pulsatile and of longer duration (5 minutes to 48 hours). The ICHD-II criteria for primary exertional headache are listed in Table 13–2.

As in cough headache, neuroimaging to rule out a posterior fossa or craniocervical junction abnormality should be undertaken in a patient presenting with new exertional headache, particularly when the headache is unilateral. In addition to unilaterality, secondary exertional headache often begins later in life, lasts longer (24 hours to weeks), and, in cases of subarachnoid hemorrhage, is associated with neurological features such as meningismus.

Other secondary causes include Chiari malformation, subdural hematoma, neoplasm (primary and metastatic), and platybasia. A "first-ever" presentation of exertional headache requires a work-up to rule out subarachnoid hemorrhage or arterial dissection (see Chapter 6).

Indomethacin is the treatment of choice in patients who frequently experience cough headache, and the sustained-release formulation (75 mg qd or bid) offers better clinical relief. A positive response to indomethacin may be seen in secondary cases and is therefore not diagnostic of primary cough headache. Other agents that have been reported to offer benefit include naproxen, acetazolamide, propanolol, methysergide, dihydroergotamine, and topiramate. In a small case series, Raskin (1995) reported that lumbar puncture with removal of 40 cc of CSF provided prompt relief.

Although our patient meets all the clinical criteria for primary cough headache, he still needs further investigations to rule out intracranial pathology. Magnetic resonance imaging of the brain should be done. If the MRI results are normal then a good treatment choice would be indomethacin 75 mg sustained release daily along with a nonnarcotic cough suppressant.

KEY POINTS TO REMEMBER

- Cough headache is symptomatic in about 40% of cases and may be the result of lesions in the posterior fossa, craniocervical junction, or CSF pathways, so neuroimaging required.
- Primary cough headache typically affects men over 40 years of age and is of short duration (1 second to 30 minutes), bilateral, and unassociated with nausea or vomiting.
- Cough headache may be precipitated by coughing, sneezing, straining, or other Valsalva maneuver.
- Treatment is with indomethacin, but lumbar puncture may also be curative.

Further Reading

Newman LC, Grosberg BM, Dodick DW. Other primary headaches. In: Silberstein SD, Lipton RB, Dodick DW (eds), Wolff's Headache and Other Head Pain, 8th ed. New York: Oxford University Press, 2008, pp 431-447.

Pasqual J. Primary cough headache. Curr Pain Headache Rep 2005;4:124-128.

Raskin NH. The cough headache syndrome: treatment. Neurology 1995;45:1784.

14 Nummular Headache

A 32-year-old accountant describes pain "right there" (indicating an area about an inch in diameter in his right parietal region) for the past 3 months. He states that the pain is nearly constant, although it waxes and wanes, and can be distracting. He says it feels like a toothache and seems to be triggered sometimes by cold air on his head or by scratching that area. He has noted some sharp "stabbing pains" in the same region and relates some unpleasant (but not necessarily painful) sensations in the general region, perhaps for an even longer time. He thinks there has not been much nausea but admits to some "queasiness" when the pain persists at higher levels. He feels certain that "there is something there" and is clearly in some emotional distress. He denies photosensitivity and has had no other pain. He does not recall recent head injury. Over-the-counter medications have not helped, and the triptan medication prescribed by his primary-care physician has been ineffective as well. His neurological examination reveals some numbness in the area of his pain but is otherwise normal.

What do you do now?

Nummular ("coin-shaped") headache (NH) is characterized by generally continuous but not usually severe pain limited to a small area of the scalp. There can be sharp pains (lancinations) superimposed upon the baseline aching pain. The parietal area seems to be the most common site. Sometimes the affected area is tender to the touch. In addition to pain, patients commonly experience decreased sensation in the area (or adjacent areas), dysesthesias (unpleasant sensation after nonnoxious stimulus), and paresthesias. Neurological examination and neuroimaging are normal. There can be spontaneous periods of remission. This headache type is not listed in the International Classification of Headache Disorders, second edition, proper but rather is a proposed defined disorder listed in the appendix (Table 14–1).

Diagnostic possibilities include intracranial mass, skull lesion, scalp infection or mass, and referred pain from a more distant head, face, or neck lesion. Computed tomography (CT) or magnetic resonance imaging (MRI) and careful assessment of the scalp and head are generally sufficient to rule these out.

Nummular headache has been termed an "epicrania" (headache due to a pain source in the scalp) and is probably a localized terminal branch neuralgia of the trigeminal nerve. Recently, Pareja et al. (2007), who first described NH, reported a series of patients with NH who had trophic changes such as hair loss and skin depression in the area of the head pain and suggested that these may herald the development of a complex regional pain syndrome (CRPS).

Treatment consists first of reassurance—that this is not a life-threatening disorder and that even though it feels like "something is there," there is no intracranial lesion. (Seeing the entirely normal CT or MR images,

TABLE 14-1   Appendix ICHD Diagnostic Criteria for Nummular Headache

A. Mild to moderate head pain fulfilling criteria B and C

B. Pain is felt exclusively in a rounded or elliptical area typically 2-6 cm in diameter

C. Pain is chronic and either continuous or interrupted by spontaneous remissions lasting weeks to months

D. Not attributed to another disorder

particularly in the vicinity of the focal pain and abnormal sensations, can be very comforting to the patient.) Non-steroidal anti-inflammatory medication seems to help patients with NH. Since the pain probably represents neuralgia, prophylactic medication helpful in other neuralgias should also be considered. Gabapentin has been used successfully, and it seems reasonable to consider other antiepileptic medications as well as tricyclic antidepressant-type medications.

Alternatively, infiltration of the sensitive area with local anesthetic may be both diagnostic and therapeutic, with pain relief sometimes lasting much longer that the action of the local anesthetic. Agents that are useful include lidocaine 1% and bupivacaine 0.25%. Many employ a 1:1 mix of both of these and inject approximately 1–2 cc into the middle of the involved region, with the patient directing the location. The addition of corticosteroids along with local anesthetic is often done but probably adds no benefit. Mathew et al. (2008) have proposed local injection of botulinum toxin for intractable cases. The possibility that NH may progress to a chronic form with features of CRPS might encourage early treatment.

KEY POINTS TO REMEMBER

- Focal head pain may be due to scalp, skull, or intracranial lesions but, when strictly localized to a coin-shaped area and associated with other sensory phenomena, may represent NH.
- Nummular headache is thought to represent focal neuralgia and, thus, may respond to antineuralgia treatment.
- Infiltration of the area of pain with local anesthetic can be therapeutic as well as diagnostic.

Further Reading

Mathew NT, Kailasam J, Meadors L. Botulinum toxin type A for the treatment of nummular headache: four case studies. Headache 2008;48:442–447.
Pareja JA, Caminero AB, Serra J, Barriga FJ, Barón M, Dobato JL, et al. Nummular headache: a coin-shaped cephalgia. Neurology 2002;58:1678–1679.
Pareja JA, Cuadrado ML, Fernández-de-las Peñas C, et al. Nummular headache with trophic changes inside the painful area. Cephalalgia 2007;28(2):186–190.

Treatment Considerations

Menstrual Headaches

A 25-year-old woman has severe migraine headaches, particularly around menses. Some of her migraines are preceded by visual aura symptoms including scintillations and scotomata, which last at most 15 minutes. She develops photo- and phonophobia, but there are no other accompaniments. Headaches last at least 24 hours and can recur over several days. She also has severe menstrual cramps and typically experiences significant moodiness prior to her menstrual periods. Both migraines and menstrual cramps have been dramatically reduced by an oral contraceptive containing both estrogen and progesterone. She is concerned about the safety of continuing this. Previous medications for migraine were ineffective except for rizatriptan, which she uses effectively for the occasional migraines she still experiences.

What do you do now?

Headache Diary

M	T	W	Th	Fr	Sa	Su
		1	2	3	4	5
6	7	8 H	9	10	11	12
13	14	15 H	16 M H	17 M	18 M H	19 M
20 M	21 M	22 M H	23	24	25	26
27	28	29	30			

				1	2 H	3 H
4	5	6	7	8	9	10
11	12	13	14 H	15	16 M H	17 M
18 M H	19 M H	20 M	21 M	22	23 H	24
25	26	27	28 H	29	30	31

FIGURE 15-1 Typical headache diary over 2 months for a patient with menstrually related migraine, with clustering of headaches around the beginning of menses as well as occasional nonmenstrual migraines, some of which could be ovulatory. M, menses; H, headache.

Menstrually related migraines (MRMs) are typical during the time period this patient describes—from 2 days prior to the onset of menses, "d–2," to the third day of flow, "d+3" (see Fig. 15–1). The majority of women with migraine, in fact, experience MRM. The headaches are generally not associated with auras, for unclear reasons. It is thought by many that it is the drop in estrogen blood levels that leads to migraine, but details as to how this trigger produces the headache are unknown. A different type of headache can occur premenstrually as part of the "premenstrual syndrome" (PMS) or "late luteal phase dysphoric disorder" (LLDD), along with fatigue, emotional lability, anxiety, etc. These headaches generally have fewer migraine features and tend to respond to different treatment. While there is some overlap between these two conditions, the patient described above seems to have MRM, as well as migraine with aura on occasion (probably nonmenstrually).

Triptans tend to be effective treatment for MRM and have even been used as "miniprophylaxis," for example, orally on a bid schedule during the vulnerable times each month. So it is not surprising that rizatriptan is of help to her, and this could be continued. Other alternatives for acute treatment are the same as those used for migraine in general—non-steroidal anti-inflammatory drugs (NSAIDs), ergot derivatives, opioids, isometheptene mucate (Midrin), and other combination medications like acetaminophen–aspirin–caffeine (although limits must be employed to prevent medication overuse headache). It is also not surprising that her estrogen–progesterone oral contraceptive (EPOC) is helping both her MRM and menstrual cramps since both conditions have been improved in this way for many women. The severe menstrual cramps she experiences may in fact be a clue that she has endometriosis, a condition comorbid with migraine and responsive to hormonal treatment. This might be worth investigation by her gynecologist. Interestingly, EPOCs and other hormonal agents are said to induce migraine headaches (either bringing on migraine for the first time or worsening pre-existing migraine). Evidence for this is weak, but many anecdotes support it in selected patients. In the case above the opposite is true, another relatively common phenomenon.

The problem here lies with the accepted belief that estrogen-containing medications should be avoided in patients with migraine with aura. Data strongly suggest that both migraine and oral contraceptives are associated with an increased risk of ischemic stroke, and patients with migraine with aura have a greater risk than women with migraine without aura (see McGregor, 2004, for a review of this). Interestingly, there are no compelling data concerning the stroke risk for older women using hormone replacement therapy. It will be important to see what this patient's headache log reveals—how frequent the headaches are, how often she does experience aura, how long it lasts, and whether any of her menstrual headaches are accompanied by aura. One suspects that virtually all of her menstrual migraines are sans aura.

So, what to do here? A good first step is always to discuss tough decisions like this with the patient. She is reluctant to make a change and for good reason—things are going well. When she understands the stroke risk, she will likely agree to try alternatives since there are some good ones. Initially, discontinuing the EPOC and seeing her gynecologist about contraceptive options, PMS, and menstrual cramps would be reasonable. Trying triptan "miniprophylaxis"—that is, daily during the vulnerable d-2 through d+3 or beyond—might be very effective, sticking with the triptan she is comfortable with. If this does not work, then NSAIDs in combination with PRN triptan use might work or perhaps institution of a prophylactic agent like topiramate, a beta-blocker, or a cyclic antidepressant might be appropriate, particularly if the headache log reveals a high frequency. (However, if the treatment for this patient's PMS ends up being a selective serotonin reuptake inhibitor, the most useful class of medication for LLDD, a cyclic antidepressant may not be the best choice.) If the choice is made to use anticonvulsant medication, it is important to warn the patient that any of these may reduce the contraceptive effectiveness of the oral contraceptive pill. If this does not work out, a try at using "phytoestrogens" (e.g., genistein and daidzein) might help the symptoms that her EPOC did. There is not much evidence yet for this, but it seems to offer benefit to some women. Magnesium at high dose either perimenstrually or continuously in a dosage of 500–600 mg daily has also been effective for some women with MRM (see Table 15–1 for a list of preventive treatment options in MRM). The ergot derivative methylergonovine (available as Methergine) can also be helpful as "miniprophylaxis," and even methysergide (Sansert) used for several days each month is considered safe enough. Vasoconstriction risks must be kept in mind, and menstrual cramping can probably be exacerbated by this class of agents. It is important to remember that triptans should not be used simultaneously with any of the ergot derivatives.

However, if the above approaches fail and this patient wants to return to hormonal treatment, it is not irresponsible to consider this as an option, considering the fact that the stroke risk in her age group, even with migraine with aura and estrogen intake, is quite low if there are no other risk factors like tobacco use, hypertension, hyperlipidemia, obesity, or diabetes. Trying a progesterone-only agent is unlikely to help migraines and, in fact, might exacerbate them. One could return to an EPOC, although the lowest dose

TABLE 15-1 **Preventive Treatment of Menstrual Migraine**

Medication Class	Examples	Dose
Triptans	Sumatriptan po	25-50 mg bid-tid d-3-d+4
	Rizatriptan po	10 mg bid d-3-d+4
	Naratriptan po	1-2.5 mg bid d-3-d+4
	Frovatriptan po	2.5 mg daily d-3-d+4
NSAIDs	Naproxen sodium	550 mg bid d-3-d+4
	Ibuprofen	400-800 mg bid d-3-d+4
Beta-blockers	Atenolol	25 mg bid or d-3-d+4
	Metoprolol	50 mg daily or d-3-d+4
Magnesium	Magnesium gluconate	500-600 mg daily
Ergots	Dihydroergotamine nasal	tid d-3-d+4
	Methylergonovine	0.2-0.4 mg tid d-3-d+4
	Methysergide (Sansert)	4 mg bid d-3-d+4
Estrogen	Estrogen + progesterone combination medication	As cyclic dose (typical for oral contraceptive pills)
	Estrogen alone—oral, transdermal	d-3-d+4 or 3-month courses
Phytoestrogens	Soy extract	Daily or d-3-d+4
Dopamine agonists	Bromocriptine	2.5 mg tid or d-3-d+4

NSAID, non-steroidal anti-inflammatory drug; d-3, 3 days prior to onset of menses; d+4, fourth day of flow.

possible would be optimal. There is some evidence for gonadotropin-releasing hormone treatment, which is probably not appropriate in this case as it leads to artificial menopause and hypogonadism. An alternative would be one of the selective estrogen receptor modulators (e.g., raloxifene), although evidence for their effectiveness in MRM is minimal. Finally, the progesterone inhibitor bromocriptine has been employed effectively for MRM but, again, is probably not appropriate here. Of note, diuretics, vitamins, and other "natural" remedies have been used for prevention of menstrual migraines but there is no evidence that they help. Hysterectomy and oophorectomy have also been proposed as successful treatments of MRM, but a lack of evidence and the potential consequences argue against them.

- Menstrual migraines are a common form of migraine, generally migraine without aura, and can be disabling.
- Focused "miniprophylaxis" treatments during the perimenstrual period can be very successful, but acute treatments are generally necessary as well, including triptans.
- Estrogenic agents are contraindicated in younger women who have migraine with aura because of postulated increased stroke risks, although their use can sometimes be justified if low doses are used and other risk factors are minimized.

Further Reading

Burke BE, Olson RD, Cusack BJ. Randomized, controlled trial of phytoestrogen in the prophylactic treatment of menstrual migraine. Biomed Pharmacother 2002;56:283-288.

Kurth T, Slomke MA, Kase CS. Migraine, headache, and the risk of stroke in women: a prospective study. Neurology 2005;64:1020-1026.

Martin V. Menstrual migraine: a review of prophylactic therapies. Curr Pain Headache Rep 2004;8:229-237.

McGregor EA. Oestrogen and attacks of migraine with and without aura. Lancet Neurol 2004;3:354-361.

Tzourio C, Tehindrazanarivelo A, Iglésias S, Alpérovitch A, Chedru F, d'Anglejan-Chatillon J, Bousser MG. Case-control study of migraine and risk of ischaemic stroke in young women. BMJ 1995;310:830-833.

Analgesic Overuse

A 36-year-old woman with chronic migraine is in your office for the first time. She has a history consistent with transformed migraines secondary to analgesic rebound. She has successfully weaned off all analgesics numerous times in the past and for prolonged periods, yet continues to suffer from daily headaches despite appropriate preventive agents. Two previous hospitalizations for treatment with intravenous dihydroergotamine resulted in relief of headaches only during the hospitalizations; headaches recurred within 2 days of discharge. Prior work-up was normal. Current medical and neurological exams are normal. Although you counsel her about acute medication limits, she asks, "Why do I need to avoid taking these medications daily? My headache frequency is exactly the same whether I take them or not, but at least I have some relief when I can treat them."

What do you do now?

This is an uncommon but not a rare occurrence in headache subspecialty practices, and it always poses a conundrum. In essence, we need to ask ourselves why treatment has failed. And if we determine that everything appropriate was done, how can we guarantee that by allowing the patient to continue to use even limited amounts of the medications there will not be dose escalation? Furthermore, what are the potential long-term consequences of daily analgesic use?

Treatment failure in headache is multifactorial. Often, the headache diagnosis is wrong, while other times the diagnosis is incomplete. Migraine may be misdiagnosed as sinus or tension-type headache; paroxysmal hemicrania may be mistaken for cluster. A more worrisome scenario occurs when a secondary headache disorder is misidentified as a primary headache. At times, the patient suffers from more than one headache type. Treating one headache type while ignoring the other will lead to an incomplete treatment response.

Other common reasons for treatment failure include inappropriate or subtherapeutic pharmacotherapy. Although the patient usually states that he or she has been prescribed all available medications, it is important to review the dosage employed, the duration of treatment, and the actual response to the therapy. Ensure that the medication was begun at a low dose, gradually increased, and continued for a proper therapeutic trial.

Frequently, patients discontinue a medication before it can be of benefit. In general, a trial of 4–6 weeks is needed to evaluate efficacy. Discuss reasons for the medication discontinuation as patients often stop a treatment inappropriately. Medication side effects may be misinterpreted as allergic reactions, or a self-limited reaction (paresthesias, sedation, etc.) is misperceived as too disabling or potentially permanent.

Very commonly, treatment failure is the result of a coexistent precipitating or exacerbating factor that has been overlooked. Issues to be explored include diet (caffeine overuse or withdrawal, artificial sweeteners, missed or irregular mealtimes), sleep patterns, stress, and hormonal status. Comorbid medical disorders such as anxiety, depression, cardiac disease, or pulmonary disease or the medications used to treat these conditions may worsen the headaches or interfere with the treatment. Most importantly, the clinician must search for medication overuse. The frequent use (daily or near daily) of acute agents, including over-the-counter medications, is the most common cause of treatment refractoriness yet is often permitted to occur. These medications induce "rebound" headache and limit the effectiveness of the migraine preventives.

The frequency of analgesic use required to produce medication overuse headache (MOH) is not clear, and there is probably a fair amount of individual variation among patients. However, an average minimum frequency is around 3 days per week. If patients keep their use of analgesics or other acute medication below this frequency, most will not fall into the MOH pattern. And use of multiple agents on different days does not exempt patients from the risk—that is, they really need to avoid *all* acute medications on 5 days per week. Medication overuse also, of course, may lead to psychological dependence, medication tolerance, and withdrawal syndromes.

Most patients with MOH can be treated on an outpatient basis. Depending on the medication, patients are either slowly weaned (for butalbital, narcotics, and caffeine-containing products) or abruptly discontinued (simple analgesics, ergots, triptans) while preventive medications are initiated. "Bridging therapies" should be employed as a stopgap measure to treat breakthrough pain. These transitional therapies, such as long-acting non-steroidal anti-inflammatory drugs (NSAIDs) like nabumetone or etodolac, meclofenamate, or the cyclooxygenase-II inhibitor celecoxib, may be used to treat acute pain flare-ups. Occasionally, a tapering course of prednisone over 10–14 days is instituted to break the pain cycle as the preventive agents are started. Severe attacks may be treated with triptans or dihydroergotamine nasal spray, but the patient must be limited to no more than two treatments weekly. If the patient is overusing caffeine-containing medications, care must be taken to slowly wean the patient from all sources of caffeine.

If the patient is overusing butalbital-containing medications in small quantities (one to five tablets daily), a reasonable approach would be to decrease the intake by one tablet per day per week. In patients whose intake is greater than five tablets daily, switching the short-acting butalbital to longer-acting phenobarbital is a better option. Using this strategy, 30 mg of phenobarbital is substituted for every 100 mg of butalbital (Fiorinal and Esgic contain 50 mg per tablet) and tapered by 15–30 mg daily. Opioids should be tapered by 10–15% every week. Clonidine 1 mg bid–tid is useful for reducing withdrawal symptoms.

These issues should be addressed and then reexplored over the course of follow-up visits. By reviewing old records and interviewing the patient (it is often very useful to reinterview the patient as if it was the initial consultation), past inadequacies may be brought into focus and new options discovered. For truly refractory patients, a second opinion can uncover clues previously overlooked.

On a first visit it is prudent to rethink or even redo the diagnostic work-up. Were all options attempted? Were dosages correct and therapeutic trials sufficiently long? Were medications used in combination and behavioral therapies employed? Were nerve blocks or other interventional techniques attempted? Usually, the savvy clinician can find treatment options that were not utilized. That the patient notes one medication only prevents or reduces her headaches suggests medication overuse. Counseling her about the detriments of medication overuse may be futile in her case in that she points out that her headaches recur soon after hospitalizations and that when going for prolonged periods without medications her headaches are unchanged. However, it might be worthwhile to attempt another inpatient admission to a center where a longer stay and a more aggressive treatment approach could be attempted (see Chapter 20).

A more difficult situation arises when the patient in question is an established one, a patient the clinician knows well and for whom all reasons for treatment unresponsiveness have been eliminated. This patient has tried medications in combination, biobehavioral and invasive therapies, and appropriate, long-duration, aggressive inpatient treatment. Despite this appropriate care and in the setting of long periods (months) of analgesic washout, she continues to suffer from ongoing, disabling headaches. Do you allow her to use daily analgesics and, if so, which ones as they differ in their potential for toxicity, abuse, and dependence?

It is the rare patient who can use daily analgesics without the subsequent need for dose escalation, but those patients do exist. In this case, I might allow the patient to continue if the daily medication was a simple analgesic, NSAID, or perhaps a combination caffeine product with or without butalbital. In these circumstances, the clinician must explain the risks and benefits of prolonged usage (cardiac, nephrotoxic, gastrointestinal, etc.), documenting this in the patient's chart with a notation that the patient is aware of the potential consequences and believes the benefits outweigh the risks. These patients need to be very closely monitored with frequent office visits and laboratory testing. On the other hand, if the patient insists on continuing a narcotic medication, an ergotamine preparation, or a triptan, I would be significantly more reticent and more than likely prohibit it.

The use of chronic opioid therapy for most patients with chronic daily headache is probably not warranted. A 5-year study of 300 patients with intractable headaches treated with long-acting opioids found that only 20% of patients were significantly improved and 40% demonstrated some evidence of noncompliance (see Saper and Lake, 2006) The authors recommended that long-term opioid therapy should be reserved for only those patients who have failed all reasonable treatment options, including hospitalization and detoxification, and who are without axis I psychiatric or personality disorders. Some have advocated the use of long-term, daily triptan use for these patients as well, based on a small open-label study.

KEY POINTS TO REMEMBER

- Refractory daily headache is usually the result of misdiagnosis, inappropriate or inadequate pharmacotherapy, or failure to identify coexisting exacerbating factors.
- Refractory daily headache commonly occurs in the setting of medication overuse.
- Refractory daily headache often requires inpatient hospitalization for detoxification and treatment.
- Chronic opioid therapy has a poor success rate and is often associated with noncompliance (dose violations, lost prescriptions, multiple prescribers).

Further Reading

Lipton RB, Silberstein SD, Saper J, Goadsby PJ. Why headache treatment fails. Neurology 2003;60:1064-1070.

Saper JR, Lake AE. Sustained opioid therapy should rarely be administered to headache patients: clinical observations, literature review, and proposed guidelines. Headache Currents 2006;3:67-70.

Sheftell FD, Rapoport AM, Tepper SJ, Bigal ME. Naratriptan in the preventive treatment of refractory transformed migraine: a prospective pilot study. Headache 2005;45:1400-1406.

17   Headaches in Pregnancy

A 20-week pregnant mother of two describes a long
history of menstrual and occasionally nonmenstrual
migrainous headaches. For the past 4 weeks, however,
she has noted a significant exacerbation of headaches
to near daily frequency with nausea. While she has not
had auras before, she recently has had some visual
changes including blurred vision and scintillating lights in
her peripheral fields around the time of migraines. The
nausea has led to a 5-pound weight loss over the past
month. Her examination is normal, although her affect
seems depressed and she looks tired. She is taking only
perinatal vitamins.

What do you do now?

Most women with migraine experience improvement, and even remission, in their headaches during pregnancy by the time of their second trimester (probably around 60%). This is even more likely in women with menstrually related migraine. But there are still many women whose headaches are unchanged (around 20%), and some experience the opposite trend—worsening of preexisting migraine, with at times disabling pain and nausea (around 20%). And some women experience their first migraine during pregnancy. Auras can occur for the first time during pregnancy as well. The case above, thus, is consistent with reports by many pregnant women (including the vagueness of the aura description). The first decision, of course, is how seriously to work up the changes in her migraine symptoms (increased frequency, aura). Gestational hypertension and preeclampsia must be ruled out, of course. (There is some evidence that eclampsia occurs earlier in women with migraine.) Without focal neurological deficits, an intracranial mass or an inflammatory or infectious process is unlikely. Cerebral venous thrombosis and pseudotumor cerebri are, however, possible; and if clinical suspicion is high or if there are even subtle neurological findings on exam, a head magnetic resonance image, magnetic resonance venogram, and lumbar puncture would be reasonable. Gadolinium is not known to be safe in pregnancy so should probably be avoided. Finally, the poorly understood syndrome of "postpartum angiopathy," also known as reversible cerebral vasoconstriction syndrome (RCVS, see Chapter 10), could be possible here and can really only be ruled out angiographically. However, RCVS is generally limited to the puerperium or late pregnancy and tends to produce multifocal neurological deficits rather than stereotypical auras.

Treatment generally begins with a concerted effort to pursue nonpharmacological treatment. Most texts emphasize the importance of reassurance and of stressing the high chance of improvement by the third trimester and, of course, following delivery. This is of small comfort to patients like the case above however. And there is the real possibility that ongoing severe migraines may themselves lead to fetal compromise, particularly if there is vomiting and dehydration. There is even some evidence that migraine is an added risk factor for stroke in pregnancy.

Relaxation training, biofeedback, and hypnotherapy can help reduce the discomfort of migraine. Even without preeclampsia, relatively risk-free magnesium supplementation at a dose of 500 mg daily may be a very effective treatment of migraine during pregnancy. Massage can be very helpful. On occasion, occipital nerve blocks or trigger point injections can be useful as well, although evidence is lacking for these interventions. Medication choices in pregnancy are limited. There are some data about drug safety in pregnancy, but sources of information differ. The U.S. Food and Drug Administration (FDA) provides a listing of relative safety, using five categories—A, B, C, D, and X (see Table 17–1). Unfortunately, very few drugs are in the "safer" categories (A and B) and many drugs are not rated. Another rating system, the Teratogen Information Service (TERIS) also provides risk categories for many drugs, from "no risk" to "high." Unfortunately, many drugs are rated "undetermined" or "unlikely." And the FDA and TERIS ratings often do not concur.

Acetaminophen is FDA category B and is useful. The addition of opioids, such as codeine, hydrocodone, oxycodone, or morphine, is controversial. They are used universally, particularly in the form of Tylenol 3; but the only opioids which are category B are oxycodone, butorphanol, and meperidine. Ibuprofen and naproxen sodium, both effective as acute treatment for many migraine patients, are FDA category B but become category D in the third trimester since non-steroidal anti-inflammatory drugs (NSAIDs) can interfere with closure of the ductus arteriosus. They may also lead to bleeding complications if used around the time of delivery. Aspirin is a category C drug in the first two trimesters but changes to category D if given

TABLE 17-1 **FDA Pregnancy Risk Categories**

Category A: Controlled human studies indicate no apparent risk to fetus. The possibility of harm to the fetus appears remote.

Category B: Either animal studies do not indicate a fetal risk or animal studies do indicate a teratogenic risk, but well-controlled human studies have failed to demonstrate the same risk.

Category C: Studies indicate teratogenic or embryocidal risks in animals, but no controlled studies have been done in women; or there are no controlled studies in animals or humans.

Category D: Positive evidence of human fetal risk, but in certain circumstances, the benefits of the drug may outweigh the risk involved.

Category X: Positive evidence of significant fetal risk, and the risk clearly outweighs any possible benefit.

in the third trimester (for the same reasons as NSAIDs). Caffeine is also category C. Triptans, particularly sumatriptan, seem to be safe during pregnancy, although this is not certain; and all are category C. Ergots, including ergotamine and dihydroergotamine are in the strictly contraindicated category X, due to their effects on implantation of the embryo, uterine blood flow, and fetal development as well as their tendency to produce uterine contractions.

Of the antiemetics, metoclopramide is in category B and is useful not only for nausea but also for antimigraine effects of its own and promotion of absorption of other analgesics. The phenothiazine antiemetics, such as prochlorperazine and promethazine, are in category C but are used when nausea and vomiting lead to dehydration and/or metabolic imbalances in pregnant women. Emetrol (phosphorylated syrup), while relatively weak, can be of use with nausea as well (Table 17–2).

Prophylactic agents, such as beta-blockers, calcium channel blockers, and cyclic antidepressants, are all category C agents (except for atenolol, which is category D) and may not even be that effective at preventing migraine during pregnancy. Prednisone is considered safe in the first trimester. Divalproex sodium (Depakote) is category D due to teratogenicity. Topiramate is in category C, but little data about its safety in pregnancy are actually available. A number of medications used to treat migraine can alter folate metabolism,

TABLE 17-2 **Selected Medications Considered Reasonably Safe for Use in Pregnancy**

Medication	FDA Category	TERIS Risk Rating
Acetaminophen	B	No risk
Ibuprofen	B (D in third trimester)	Minimal
Naproxen	B (D in third trimester)	Undetermined
Oxycodone	B (D near term)	
Magnesium	B	Unlikely
Metoclopramide	B	Unlikely
Prednisone	C in first trimester, less clear in second/third trimesters	Minimal
Promethazine	C	None

TERIS, Teratogen Information Service.

so supplementing with 0.4 mg folate daily is advisable when using daily medications.

In the above case, there are a number of factors which would suggest an aggressive approach to headaches, including headache frequency and severity, nausea and vomiting, weight loss, and depression. Diagnostic evaluation should be done, guided by careful monitoring of exams as well as response to treatment. Antinauseant medication should be employed, and both acute and perhaps preventive treatment should be instituted. And to allay the patient's fears, detailed empathetic discussion of risks and benefits must be done.

KEY POINTS TO REMEMBER

- While migraines improve during pregnancy for most women, there are many cases of the opposite, sometimes accompanied by severe nausea and vomiting.
- Diagnostic suspicion should be high with any change in headache pattern, although most headaches will be generally benign.
- Nonpharmacological therapy can help migraines in pregnancy, but judicious supplementation with pharmaceutical treatments is reasonable, particularly in severe cases.

Further Reading

Briggs GB, Yaffe SJ, Freeman RK. Drugs in Pregnancy and Lactation: A Reference Guide to Fetal and Neonatal Risk, 7th ed. Philadelphia: Lippincott Williams & Wilkins, 2005.

Cantu C, Barinagarrementeria F. Cerebral venous thrombosis associated with pregnancy and puerperium. Review of 67 cases. Stroke 1993;24;1880-1884.

Silberstein SD. Headaches in pregnancy. Neurol Clin 2004;22:727-756.

18 Hemicrania Continua

A 38-year-old woman with a 5-year history of daily headaches presents for an initial consultation. She reports that she suffers from a strictly right-sided headache of varying intensity that waxes and wanes throughout the day. She denies nausea and vomiting but reports that, when severe, the headache is associated with phonophobia and congestion of the right nostril. She has failed to respond to standard antimigraine preventions and notes that sumatriptan and almotriptan offer minimal or no benefit. Her neurological exam is normal, as are the three recent head magnetic resonance images that she brings to the visit. She is currently taking an H_2-blocker because her recent endoscopy revealed multiple gastric erosions from overuse of aspirin.

What do you do now?

This patient has very bad luck. She is suffering from hemicrania continua (HC), a disabling headache condition, and multiple gastric erosions, which prohibits prescribing the treatment of choice. Hemicrania continua is an underrecognized, primary headache disorder and a common cause of refractory, unilateral, chronic daily headache. The disorder demonstrates a marked female preponderance, with a female to male ratio of approximately 2:1. The age at onset ranges from 11 to 58 years.

Clinically, HC is characterized by a unilateral, continuous headache of mild to moderate intensity. Patients usually describe this baseline discomfort as dull, aching, or pressing; and it is not associated with other symptoms. The pain is maximal in the ocular, temporal, and maxillary regions. Superimposed upon this background discomfort, exacerbations of more severe pain, lasting 20 minutes to several days, are experienced by the majority of sufferers. Although significantly more intense than the baseline pain, these painful exacerbations never reach the level experienced by cluster headache sufferers. During these flare-ups, one or more autonomic symptoms (ptosis, conjunctival injection, lacrimation, and nasal congestion) occur ipsilateral to the pain. These exacerbations may occur at any time and frequently awaken the patient from sleep. Migrainous symptoms, such as nausea, vomiting, photophobia, and phonophobia, may also accompany the exacerbations of pain. Many patients report primary stabbing headaches (stabs and jabs) and a feeling of sand or an eyelash in the affected eye (foreign body sensation). Most patients experience strictly unilateral headaches without side shift, although three patients in whom attacks alternated sides and three bilateral cases have been described.

Two temporal profiles of HC exist: an episodic form, with distinct headache phases separated by pain-free remissions, and a chronic form, in which headaches persist without remissions.

Often, HC is misdiagnosed by clinicians unfamiliar with the disorder. If the physician focuses on the ipsilateral autonomic features that accompany the painful exacerbations, the disorder may be incorrectly diagnosed as cluster headache. Similarly, by focusing on the associated photophobia, phonophobia, nausea, and vomiting that may occur during exacerbations, HC may be misdiagnosed as migraine. It is distinguished from cluster and migraine by the presence of a continuous baseline headache of mild to moderate severity; neither the ipsilateral autonomic features of cluster nor the associated phenomena typically reported with migraine accompany this baseline pain.

Organic mimics of HC have been reported to occur in association with a mesenchymal tumor involving the sphenoid bone, clinoid process, and skull base.

Indomethacin is the treatment of choice for HC, and response to therapy with indomethacin is required by the *International Classification of Headache Disorders*, second edition (ICHD-II), criteria for establishing the diagnosis. Therapy is usually initiated at a dose of 25 mg tid and increased to 50 mg tid in 1 week if there is no response or only partial benefit. Headache resolution is usually prompt, occurring within 1–2 days after the effective dosage is reached, although response may take as long as 2 weeks. Maintenance with doses ranging 25–100 mg usually suffices; however, at times doses as high as 300 mg daily may be required.

Dosage adjustments are occasionally necessary to treat the clinical fluctuations that are sometimes seen with HC. Nighttime dosing with sustained-release indomethacin often prevents nocturnal exacerbations. During the active headache cycle, patients report that skipping or even delaying doses of indomethacin may result in the prompt reemergence of symptoms. The gastrointestinal side effects of indomethacin can be mitigated with antacids, misoprostol, or histamine H_2 receptor antagonists. These agents should always be considered for those patients requiring long-term therapy. Although the ICHD-II requires indomethacin responsiveness as a diagnostic criterion, other agents have been reported to induce a partial response. These include naproxen, paracetamol, paracetamol with caffeine, ibuprofen, piroxicam, rofecoxib (no longer available), celecoxib, melatonin, and topiramate.

Since our patient has multiple gastric erosions, the use of indomethacin or other non-steroidal anti-inflammatory drugs is contraindicated. In her case and for other patients in whom these agents are ineffective or prohibited, treatment with either melatonin or topiramate should be tried. Melatonin should be initiated at a dose of 3 mg at bedtime and can be increased by 3 mg every 3–5 nights, up to a maximum dosage of 24 mg nightly. Topiramate is dosed in HC as it is in the treatment of migraine. After her erosions heal and if she fails to respond optimally to melatonin or topiramate, treatment with indomethacin and one or more of the gastric protective agents may be employed, with the permission and supervision of her gastroenterologist.

Further Reading

Brighina F, Palermo A, Cosentino G, Fierro B. Prophylaxis of hemicrania continua: two new cases effectively treated with topiramate. Headache 2007;47:441-443.

Goadsby PJ, Lipton RB. A review of paroxysmal hemicranias, SUNCT syndrome and other short-lasting headaches with autonomic feature, including new cases. Brain 1997;120:193-209.

Newman LC, Lipton RB, Solomon S. Hemicrania continua: ten new cases and a review of the literature. Neurology 1994;44:2111-2114.

Peres MFP, Silberstein SD, Nahmias S, Shechter AL, Youssef I, Rozen TD, Young WB. Hemicrania continua is not that rare. Neurology 2001;57:948-951.

Rozen TD. Melatonin responsive hemicrania continua. Headache 2006;46:1203-1209.

Sjaastad O, Spierings ELH. Hemicrania continua: another headache absolutely responsive to indomethacin. Cephalalgia 1980;4:65-70.

Trigeminal Neuralgia

A 78-year-old woman diagnosed with trigeminal neuralgia describes lancinating and aching pain in her right cheek, upper teeth, and nostril for the past 8 months. Pain is sometimes brought on by chewing or swallowing, and there is radiation of pain to the ear and throat on occasion. She had an initial response to carbamazepine, but this, despite increasing to high doses, has lost effectiveness. Neither baclofen nor pregabalin has been helpful. The pain is interfering with sleep, and she has several sudden stabs of pain while in your office. Past medical history is remarkable for unstable angina, for which she uses nitroglycerine.

What do you do now?

Trigeminal neuralgia (TN) is not uncommon in the elderly. It is a bit more common in women and tends to involve the second and/or third divisions of the trigeminal nerve predominantly. Typically, the pain is brief, "knifelike" (i.e., lancinating), severe, and often triggered by some sensory stimulus in a "trigger zone," which can be in the territory of the pain or nearby. Triggers include chewing, swallowing, washing the face, shaving, brushing the teeth, or even feeling a breeze on the face. The pain sometimes causes a sudden facial muscle spasm, which can look like a facial tic (hence the name "tic douloureux"). Sometimes the pain persists between attacks. Exam is generally normal, but subtle facial numbness can be found in some patients.

Some cases of TN ("secondary TN") are due to compression or irritation of the trigeminal nerve by a tumor, meningeal infectious process, demyelinating lesion around the trigeminal root entry zone, or zoster infection of the nerve. When these secondary causes are ruled out, compression of the trigeminal nerve by an arterial loop has been postulated to be the cause; and while clear examples of this have been seen in neuroimaging and in the operating room, this is still controversial. Some cases of TN overlap into the syndrome of glossopharyngeal neuralgia (GN), described as similar lancinations but in the throat, posterior tongue, and ear, triggered by swallowing. Also occurring in the older age groups, GN is even more likely than TN to be due to a mass lesion—presumably somewhere along the courses of the glossopharyngeal or vagus nerve.

Differential diagnosis of TN includes dental disease, sinus disease, cluster headache, giant cell arteritis, SUNCT (short-lasting, unilateral, neuralgiform headache attacks with conjunctival injection and tearing) syndrome, postherpetic neuralgia, and primary stabbing headache ("jabs and jolts"). The above case seems to share features of both TN and GN (the two can actually coexist in approximately 10% of cases), so a search for secondary causes should be undertaken, with magnetic resonance imaging (MRI) of the head prior to and following gadolinium infusion to rule out a brainstem or skull base mass lesion. If this is normal, a lumbar puncture might be considered, to rule out an infectious or inflammatory etiology such as nonbacterial meningitis, sarcoidosis, or Lyme disease. Erythrocyte sedimentation rate should be done as well as a thorough dental evaluation (see Table 19–1 for a list of the common secondary causes of TN).

TABLE 19-1 **Secondary Causes of Trigeminal Neuralgia**

Dental root disease
Brainstem neoplasm—meningioma, metastatic tumor
Meningeal infection—fungal, Lyme, syphilis
Sarcoidosis
Multiple sclerosis—brainstem plaque
Postherpetic neuralgia of the trigeminal nerve

When work-up fails to reveal a secondary cause of TN, medical therapy should be instituted (See Table 19–2). Carbamazepine is the most likely agent to help, which unfortunately has lost its effectiveness in this case. Gabapentin can be helpful, as can other anticonvulsants including lamotrigine, phenytoin, oxcarbazepine, and pregabalin. Valproate and topiramate have been proposed, but evidence for their efficacy is scant. The evidence for baclofen's use in TN is good. Cyclic antidepressants, such as amitriptyline and nortriptyline, have been used effectively in many cases. Neuroleptic medications such as chlorpromazine have helped certain patients as well. Clonazepam has been reported to help some patients. Combining medications from any of these categories helps some patients for whom monotherapy has failed. Tolerability and medication interactions limit the use of all of these options, particularly in the elderly; but careful dosage adjustment may allow titration to effective doses, even when two or three medications are used simultaneously. Medications that work well for TN tend to also work in GN.

Surgical options for treating intractable TN fall into three categories: (*1*) procedures performed on the peripheral branches of the trigeminal nerve, (*2*) trigeminal gangliolysis, and (*3*) surgical decompression of the trigeminal nerve as it passes near the brainstem. Beneficial local blockade of one or more branches of the trigeminal nerve may predict success with more permanent blockade of these branches or of the trigeminal ganglion itself. By themselves, peripheral procedures do not seem to provide long-term relief. Gangliolysis is generally well tolerated and can be done percutaneously using radiofrequency, glycerol, or a balloon microcompression apparatus. The most widely studied is percutaneous radiofrequency trigeminal gangliolysis, which seems to help at least 90% of patients. Unfortunately, pain recurs in many (20%–30%). Microvascular decompression of the trigeminal nerve is done

TABLE 19-2   Pharmacologic Treatment of Trigeminal Neuralgia

Medication	Typical Effective Dosage
Carbamazepine (Tegretol)	100-400 mg tid po
Gabapentin (Neurontin)	300-1,200 mg tid po
Pregabalin (Lyrica)	100-200 mg tid po
Lamotrigine (Lamictal)	200-400 mg daily po
Phenytoin (Dilantin)	100 mg tid po
Baclofen	10-40 mg tid po
Amitriptyline	10-150 mg qhs po
Nortriptyline	10-75 mg qhs po
Clonazepam (Klonopin)	0.5-1 mg tid

via a suboccipital craniotomy and aims to identify a compressive vascular loop and to introduce spacing material between it and the trigeminal nerve. In the hands of experienced surgeons, this procedure has a low mortality rate (<1%) and a high success rate (long-term pain relief up to 80%).

In the case above, aggressive treatment is certainly indicated. The fact that she responded for some time to carbamazepine is actually a hopeful sign, and a good first step might be to try gabapentin, advancing the dose as tolerated. Nortriptyline might be a good adjunct agent, and clonazepam might be another, although all three have the potential to lead to adverse effects. Gabapentin can cause cognitive dysfunction, always difficult in an elderly patient. Nortriptyline can lead to tachycardia and/or prolong the Q–T interval, so electrocardiographic monitoring is important. This drug can also cause dry mouth, constipation, and possibly urine retention. Clonazepam (Klonopin) can also cause mental status changes and sedation. If this approach fails, percutaneous gangliolysis might be appropriate here because of its overall safety (no general anesthesia required).

KEY POINTS TO REMEMBER

- Trigeminal neuralgia is not uncommon in the elderly population.
- The differential diagnosis of TN is broad.

Continued

- A number of secondary causes of TN exist, so brain MRI is generally indicated.
- Both TN and GN can actually coexist in approximately 10% of cases.
- Medical treatment of TN is usually successful, with polypharmacy sometimes necessary; but this can be limited by adverse effects and medical interactions.
- Surgical options include the relatively noninvasive gangliolytic procedures.

Further Reading

Brisman R. Surgical treatment of trigeminal neuralgia. Semin Neurol 1997;17(4):367-372.

Mauskop A. Trigeminal neuralgia (tic douloureux). In: Levin M, Ward TN (eds), Head, Neck and Facial Pain. Columbus, OH: Anadem, 2006.

Nurmikko TJ, Eldridge PR. Trigeminal neuralgia–pathophysiology, diagnosis and current treatment. Br J Anaesthesiol 2001;87:117-132.

Emergency Department and Inpatient Management

A 36-year-old woman with unremitting headaches, unresponsive to several interventions by her primary-care physician, goes to the emergency department, where even intramuscular (IM) meperidine is only partially effective. Her exam was normal, but head computed tomography (CT) was done, which is likewise 100% normal. She refuses to leave the emergency department and is admitted to your service. History is unremarkable. She had migraines in her twenties, which have progressed over the past several years to daily headaches and have led to her use of four to eight butalbital-acetaminophen-caffeine (Fioricet) tablets on a daily basis. She is in tears, demanding more Fioricet and criticizing her primary-care physician for limiting her use of it.

What do you do now?

The approach to acute headache in the emergency room setting must include both diagnostic and treatment concerns. Deciding about the need for neuroimaging (CT, magnetic resonance imaging) and lumbar puncture will depend upon the presence of history and examination "red flags" (see Table 10–1). Once serious secondary causes of acute headache are ruled out, treatment can proceed. Commonly, emergency room physicians will begin with the parenteral non-steroidal anti-inflammatory drug (NSAID) ketorolac (Toradol) along with a parenteral antiemetic (e.g., promethazine 25 mg IM) if nausea is significant. If pain persists, intravenous dihydroergotamine (DHE) 1 mg or subcutaneous sumatriptan 6 mg might be very helpful since most patients with acute severe headache have migraine. Before giving DHE or sumatriptan, ensure that the patient has not taken ergots or triptans at home prior to arriving in the emergency department. These medications must not be given within 24 hours of each other. Intravenous magnesium has been used effectively in some patients at a dose of 1–4 g, via slow intravenous infusion. If this is insufficient, addition of parenteral opioid medication may be necessary, although high doses are often required. Options include meperidine 50–150 mg and morphine 2–10 mg. Meperidine is used widely but is probably not as effective as morphine and can lead to toxicity (due to its long-acting metabolite normeperidine) if used repeatedly.

Patients with frequent severe headaches often overuse acute therapies. There are many risks in doing this, including medication overuse headache, previously referred to as "rebound" headache, defined as escalation of headaches resulting from frequent use of acute medications (see Chapter 16). Medication overuse headache can occur with simple analgesics (aspirin, acetaminophen, NSAIDs), combination analgesics containing caffeine with or without butalbital, narcotics, ergots, and triptans.

Inpatient treatment of medication overuse headache is indicated in certain situations (Table 20–1). Upon admission and in the absence of contraindications, the patient can be started on treatment with intravenous DHE while being tapered off the overused medication. Patients who are overusing butalbital-containing medications in small amounts (1–10 tablets daily) should be gradually weaned off the medication. A good approach, as outlined in Chapter 16, would be to switch the short-acting butalbital to longer-acting phenobarbital. Using this strategy, 30 mg of phenobarbital is substituted for every 100 mg of butalbital (Fiorinal and Esgic contain 50 mg per tablet) and tapered by 15–30 mg daily. When patients are using these medications in higher doses (more than 10 tablets daily) or if their true intake is in doubt, an oral phenobarbital load has been shown to be a safe and effective option for withdrawing patients (see Loder and Biondi, 2003). In this method, all short-acting butalbital compounds are discontinued on the first hospital day. The patient is given phenobarbital 120 mg po hourly. Patients are evaluated

TABLE 20-1 Indications for Inpatient Treatment of Medication Overuse Headache

Headaches that interfere or disrupt activities of daily living
Chronic daily headache unresponsive to outpatient therapies
Comorbid medical or psychiatric illness
Polypharmacy
Headache complicated by drug overuse

TABLE 20-2 Protocol for Oral Phenobarbital Loading

Loading Protocol
1. At 6:00 a.m. on the first day of the protocol, all short-acting butalbital medications are discontinued. The patient is to stay at complete bed rest, and fall precautions are initiated.
2. A baseline score on the rating scale (see below) is obtained at 7:00 a.m., and the patient is administered 120 mg phenobarbital orally.
3. At each hour following the first dose, the patient is reevaluated using the rating scale. If the score is lower than 8, a dose of 120 mg phenobarbital is given orally.
4. Reevaluation and redosing are repeated hourly until the score reaches 8 or more, at which point no more phenobarbital is given.
5. Vital signs are obtained at regular intervals until the patient is reliably alert.
6. Patient remains at strict bed rest with fall precautions until cleared by physician.

Rating Scale
1. Patient evaluated in each of the following categories before first dose.
2. Reassess every hour.
3. Discontinue phenobarbital when score is 8 or more.

(Continued)

TABLE 20-2 CONTINUED

Categories

A. Nystagmus
   1. None
   2. Present in lateral gaze
   3. Easily elicited and sustained
   4. Coarse and sustained

B. Dysarthria
   1. Absent
   2. Minor slurring
   3. Moderate slurring
   4. Severe slurring, unintelligible

C. Ataxia
   1. Absent
   2. Mildly unsteady tandem gait
   3. Moderately unsteady regular gait
   4. Needs support on regular gait

D. Drowsiness
   1. Alert
   2. Awake but drowsy
   3. Asleep but easily arousable
   4. Asleep but difficult to arouse

E. Emotional lability
   1. Normal, as before loading dose
   2. Some mood change
   3. Obvious mood change
   4. Uninhibited, mood swings

Source: Loder and Biondi (2003).

every hour (Table 20–2) and are continued on phenobarbital until they reach set clinical parameters, at which point the phenobarbital is discontinued.

The standard DHE protocol involves pretreatment for each dose with metoclopramide 10 mg in 50 cc D5W over 30 minutes. A test dose of DHE 0.5 mg IV in 50 cc normal saline (NS) over 15 minutes or slowly pushed over 2 minutes is given, and treatment is continued depending on response: If headache persists and no nausea occurs, one can give DHE 0.5 mg 1 hour after the first dose and then 0.5–1.0 mg every 8 hours. If headache and nausea persist, metoclopramide can be increased to 20 mg and/or subsequent DHE doses can be decreased to 0.25 mg. If headache and nausea improve,

DHE 0.5 mg every 8 hours is continued until the headache is eliminated. Then, DHE should be continued every 12 hours for two or three doses to ensure that the cycle is broken. All patients should have standing orders for diphenhydramine in case they develop akathisia or dystonic reactions from the metoclopramide. If these symptoms develop, metoclopramide should be discontinued and pretreatment with trimethobenzamide, promethazine, ondansetron, or granisetron should be initiated.

If DHE is unhelpful or if there are contraindications to its use, other inpatient treatment options include dexamethasone 10 mg IV stat, then 4 mg every 6 hours for 1–2 days; ketorolac 30–60 mg IM or IV every 8 hours PRN for a maximum of 3 days; chlorpromazine 0.1 mg/kg IV every 6 hours; or valproate sodium 500–800 mg in 50 cc NS IV every 8 hours. Importantly, chlorpromazine may induce hypotension, so it is imperative to ensure that the patient is well hydrated prior to intravenous administration. When valproate sodium is used, patients should have periodic blood tests to monitor liver function. Patients who are taking topiramate for migraine prevention in general should not be given IV valproate sodium as the combination may induce hepatic encephalopathy. Patients on a phenobarbital taper (as above) should also not be given IV valproate sodium because of the drug interactions. These agents may also be used to supplement DHE in patients with incomplete response.

Most patients with headaches intractable enough to require hospital admission will respond to one of these approaches. The rare patients who do not probably require referral to a headache treatment center, where a multidisciplinary team approach can be employed, including psychological, anesthesiological, and physical medicine measures.

KEY POINTS TO REMEMBER

- The emergency room approach to headache includes diagnostic and treatment decision making, often simultaneously. Once secondary headaches are excluded, there are a number of effective treatment options.

Continued

- Treatment of medication overuse headache is sometimes best done on an inpatient basis, particularly when the headache is due to medications that may be dangerous to withdraw on an outpatient basis or if other psychosocial factors dictate.
- Inpatient headache treatment tools include parenteral DHE, dexamethasone, ketorolac, chlorpromazine, and valproate sodium.

Further Reading

American College of Emergency Physicians. Clinical policy. Critical issues in the evaluation and management of patients presenting to the emergency department with acute headache. Ann Emerg Med 2002;39(1):108-122.

Diener HC, Katsarava Z. Medication overuse headache. Curr Med Res Opin 2001; 17:s17–s21.

Krymchantowski AV, Moreira PF. Out-patient detoxification in chronic migraine: comparison of strategies. Cephalalgia 2003;23:982-993.

Loder E, Biondi D. Oral phenobarbital loading: a safe and effective method of withdrawing patients with headache from butalbital compounds. Headache 2003;43:904-909.

Raskin NH. Repetitive intravenous dihydroergotamine as therapy for intractable migraine. Neurology 1986;36:995-997.

Occipital Neuralgia

Last winter, a 44-year-old teacher, while walking down icy steps at school, slipped, fell backward, and struck her occiput. She did not lose consciousness. She experienced moderately severe global headache and neck pain for the next 2 days and then felt well. Approximately 2–3 weeks later she began to experience brief episodes of sharp pain in the right occipital area, which seemed unrelated to movement or position.

This pain was not associated with any other symptoms. Pain radiated to the right temple and, at times, to the right eye. After several more weeks, she began to experience aching pain in the same area (right occipitotemporal), and this has persisted on a virtually daily basis since then. She finds that pressure on the back of her head seems to intensify the pain, and she has had to adjust her sleeping position to avoid contact in the right and posterior areas of her scalp. She is otherwise asymptomatic. Her neurological exam is normal, as is head magnetic resonance imaging (MRI). There is some tenderness in her occiput and some tightness and tenderness in her posterior cervical muscles. She is using a large number of ibuprofen and acetaminophen tablets monthly (but she cannot specify the quantity). These analgesics serve only to dull the pain somewhat. Amitriptyline, methocarbamol, and cyclobenzaprine have not helped. She bursts into tears while relating this history.

What do you do now?

This patient may have posttraumatic headache (see Chapter 28), but her history and exam suggest occipital neuralgia (ON). This condition, also referred to as "occipital neuritis," is not uncommon after posterior head trauma, presumably due to the propensity for damage to the relatively superficial greater occipital nerve (GON), which can easily be compressed against the skull. Neuromas can form on the nerve, but this is not consistent. In some cases, it is postulated that the actual site of damage or lesion is the C2 nerve root (which essentially becomes the GON distally).

Diagnosis of ON is made on the basis of (*1*) a history of posterior head trauma, (*2*) tenderness of the occipital nerve, and (*3*) resolution of pain by local anesthetic block of the GON. Like trigeminal neuralgia (TN), ON's key feature is lancinating pain emanating from the involved nerve. As with TN, persistent aching pain is also common, particularly as the process becomes chronic. This may be related to central sensitization. Radiation to temporal and even more anterior structures, like the ipsilateral eye, is thought to be due to the convergence that occurs at the spinal cord level between nociceptive afferents from anterior head and posterior head regions (trigeminal and upper cervical roots).

Differential diagnosis includes a number of primary and secondary headache disorders: postherpetic neuralgia involving the C2 root or GON; scalp infection or other inflammation; pathological processes involving the upper cervical spine, such as rheumatoid arthritis (or other arthropathy), spinal tumors, or infections of the upper cervical spine; and disorders of the craniocervical junction or posterior cranial fossa, including masses or infections and Chiari I malformation (see Chapter 7). Occasionally, temporal arteritis (see Chapter 5) can mimic some features of ON, and migraine can manifest with occipital pain. Investigation of patients like this therefore should usually include inspection of the scalp in the region, cervical spinal examination, imaging of the cervical spine (plain X-ray series might be sufficient), erythrocyte sedimentation rate, and MRI of the head, which should include the craniocervical junction region.

The most useful initial treatment of ON is also diagnostic—anesthetic blockade of the GON. The technique of GON block is relatively simple (see Figure 21–1). The trunk of the GON is located approximately one-third of the distance on a line from the external occipital protuberance to the center of the mastoid. It is adjacent to the occipital artery and can be located by palpating for this artery. Injection of approximately 1–2 cc of 0.25% bupivacaine or 1% lidocaine (or a mixture of the two) in the area of the GON should be sufficient. The GON innervates the scalp from the level of the external occipital protuberance to the vertex on each side, so it is possible to assess the degree of anesthesia by simple sensory testing in the area. The lesser occipital nerve is sometimes involved in the production of pain and can also be blocked with a similar technique and agents (see Figure 21–1).

It seems that clinical benefit is greatest when the area of anesthesia achieved includes the area of the patient's pain. The anesthesia should last for several hours (1–2 hours with lidocaine and more like 4–6 hours for bupivacaine). The surprising thing about this technique is that it can provide relief for patients for much longer—days to weeks or even longer. With this patient's history of heavy use of non-steroidal anti-inflammatory drugs (NSAIDs), bleeding may complicate the procedure (NSAIDs inhibit

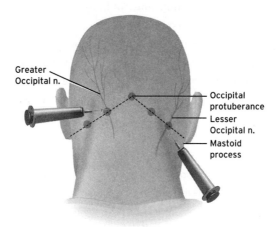

FIGURE 21-1 Technique for performing greater and lesser occipital nerve (GON, LON) blocks. For GON block, the needle tip is inserted approximately one-third of the distance on a line from the external occipital protuberance to the center of the mastoid. For LON block, the injection site is lateral and inferior to the GON site. (Used by permission of Oxford University Press, *Wolff's Headache and Other Head Pain*, Silberstein et al., 2007.)

platelet aggregation and prolong bleeding time). Other risks of GON blocks include local site infection (rare) and effects of inadvertent intravascular injection such as light-headedness, tinnitus, anxiety, loss of consciousness, or seizure (unusual because of the low dose of anesthetic and generally easy to avoid by pulling back on the plunger prior to injecting).

If local anesthesia of the GON is effective but pain returns, subsequent GON blocks may prove longer-lasting. One can add a corticosteroid, such as triamcinolone, although this has not been shown to be any more effective than the local anesthetic agents by themselves. If this is not successful, implantation of a GON stimulator might be warranted. This is costly and carries some minor morbidity risk, but in many cases the benefits are clearly worth the expense and risks. If pain is refractory, further work-up may be appropriate, such as MRI of the cervical spine to search for pathology; C2 root block may also be worth trying. This procedure is a bit more challenging and should be performed under fluoroscopy by trained personnel. However, it can be very effective.

Oral prophylactic medication can help some patients. If the cause of the pain is postherpetic neuralgia, carbamazepine, gabapentin, or pregabalin might be of help. In idiopathic ON, tricyclic antidepressants, anticonvulsants, clonazepam, and NSAIDs have all been helpful in some patients. Muscle relaxants have not proven effective, despite the tender muscle spasm seen in many patients.

KEY POINTS TO REMEMBER

- Occipital neuralgia presents with stabbing pain in the occipital region but can also include more persistent aching pain.
- There may be no antecedent history of trauma to the nerve, but presentation should include some tenderness over the GON trunk.
- Differential diagnosis includes pathology in the region of the upper cervical spine, craniocervical junction, or posterior fossa.
- Block of the GON is often both diagnostic and therapeutic.

Further Reading

Anthony M. Headache and the greater occipital nerve. Clin Neurol Neurosurg 1992;94:297-301.

Ashkenazi A, Levin M. Nerve blocks and other procedures for headache. In: Silberstein SD, Lipton RB, Dalessio DJ. Wolff's Headache and Other Head Pain, 8th ed. New York: Oxford University Press, 2007.

Bogduk N. Role of anesthesiologic blockade in headache management. Curr Pain Headache Rep 2004;8(5):399-403.

Goadsby PJ, Bartsch T, Dodick DW. Occipital nerve stimulation for headache: mechanisms and efficacy. Headache 2008;48(2):313-318.

Silberstein SD, Lipton RB, Dodick DW (eds). Wolff's Headache and Other Head Pain, 8th ed. New York: Oxford University Press, 2007, p.769.

22 Headache Recurrence

It is the first visit for this 27-year-old man, who describes
a several-year history of migraine without aura. He
reports that his headaches occur three or four times
monthly but resolve within 2 hours with 5 mg of oral
zolmitriptan. He takes no other medication and has
no other significant medical history. As you write his
prescription refill, he asks for a medication override,
allowing him 18 tablets per month. Perplexed, you
inquire why he needs so many pills if he only gets three
or four headaches monthly. He tells you that although
the medication works quickly, the headache returns
either later that day or sometime the next day; this cycle
continues for 4 days.

What do you do now?

This case illustrates several important issues. First, it demonstrates the need for clinicians to inquire about the number of headache *days* rather than the number of *headaches* per month. Second, this case highlights the need for the clinician to ask about treatment success and to define success in specific terms. A good benchmark for success would be that one dose of the acute medication terminates the headache and associated symptoms of the migraine attack within 2 hours and that the headache does not return within the next 24 hours.

There are many reasons for treatment refractoriness (see Chapter 16). Our patient suffers from headache recurrence, the return of an episodic headache during the same migraine attack following the use of an acute treatment. Approximately 20% of triptan users experience a recurrence of their headache 2–24 hours after dosing. For most patients, repeating the same medication will afford relief. In other patients, like the one described in our case, this cycle can linger for several days with a waxing and waning course. In these instances, the clinician has several options: ensuring that the patient treats the headache early in the attack (within the first 40 minutes of headache onset), that the optimal dose is employed (the highest available dose of the triptan nearly always has a better response), and that the proper formulation is used. Specifically, oral medications should be avoided in patients with vomiting; nasal spray and parenteral formulations are ideal in this setting. If these measures do not optimize the therapeutic response, additional options include switching to a different triptan (naratriptan and frovatriptan have a lower recurrence rate) or adding a non-steroidal anti-inflammatory drug (NSAID), such as naproxen sodium, to the triptan at headache onset. A new combination product containing sumatriptan 85 mg and naproxen sodium 500 mg became available in the United States in 2008.

Despite the fact that triptans have revolutionized the acute treatment of migraine, they are not a panacea. As many as 40% of all migraine attacks and a quarter of all patients do not respond to the eight currently available triptan formulations. Triptan nonresponse is defined by failure to successfully treat an acute attack on three separate occasions with three different agents and subcutaneous sumatriptan. For triptan nonresponders, trials of dihydroergotamine, parenterally or intranasally, should be employed.

Lastly, this case may represent a potential candidate for preventive therapy. Just as poor communication between the patient and clinician can lead to underestimating the disability induced by migraine, so too can it lead to the underutilization of preventive medications. Lipton et al. (2007) reported that approximately 40% of migraine sufferers are candidates for migraine prevention but only 13% actually receive treatment. If our patient's headaches continue to be inadequately controlled by the measures discussed above, he should be prescribed a preventive therapy.

KEY POINTS TO REMEMBER

- Headache recurrence refers to the return of an episodic headache during the same migraine attack following the use of an acute treatment.
- Headache recurrence occurs in approximately 20% of triptan users and usually responds to an additional dose of the same medication.
- Headache recurrence may be lessened by
  - Treating early in the attack
  - Using the highest dose of the triptan
  - Avoiding oral formulations in patients who vomit
  - Switching to another triptan
  - Adding an NSAID to the triptan
  - Switching to dihydroergotamine

Further Reading

Ferrari MD, Roon KI, Lipton RB, Goadsby P. Oral triptans (serotonin 5HT (1B/1D) agonists) in acute migraine treatment: a meta-analysis of 53 trials. Lancet 2001;358:1688-1675.

Lipton RB, Bigal ME, Diamond M, et al. Migraine prevalence, disease burden, and the need for preventive therapy. Neurology 2007;68:343-349.

Visser WH, Jaspers N, de Vriend RMH, Ferrari MD. Risk factors for headache recurrence after sumatriptan; a study of 366 migraine patients. Cephalalgia 1996;16:264-269.

23 Headache and Allergy

A 35-year-old woman complains of daily headaches, which build in intensity through the morning and generally only resolve when she lies down to go to sleep each evening. She reports that she has "taken everything out of my diet" (meat, sugar, additives, alcohol, caffeine) and that this helped somewhat. She believes that she has food and environmental allergies and has tried to avoid as many of these as she can. Skin testing confirmed several of these. She has lactose intolerance and avoids dairy products. She wonders if she has celiac disease. She has seen many physicians, nutritionists, chiropractors, massage therapists, an acupuncturist, and now a craniosacral therapist. No traditional medical therapy "has ever worked," and many medications have led to "horrible" side effects. She refuses to take any pills because of her past experience and because of potential allergens in the colorings in their coatings. The only medication she uses is Excedrin Migraine, which she takes daily, between four and eight tablets.

What do you do now?

This patient with chronic daily headache (CDH)—that is, headaches on more than 15 days per month—seems to be telling you that she is not willing to try any medications whatsoever. However, she does use the acetaminophen–aspirin–caffeine combination, which, by the way, does contain possibly allergenic colorings and excipients. It is also almost certainly leading to medication overuse headache, which can be hard to prove and even more difficult to reverse if she is unwilling to take any prophylactic medications. This is a tough spot for both the patient and the clinician.

A good first step, as always, is to do what one can to confirm the presumptive diagnosis of primary headache (which type is hard to determine at this point) with medication overuse–induced CDH. Thorough neurological, head and neck, dental, and general exams should be done. Magnetic resonance imaging of the head will rule out structural lesions, and basic metabolic and hematological screening will rule out such issues as thyroid disease and anemia. Celiac disease, of course, can cause headaches; but usually gastrointestinal symptoms predominate. Serological endomysial antibody screening is a good noninvasive tool, but the gold standard for the diagnosis of celiac disease remains histological confirmation with intestinal biopsy. Another option is to try restriction of wheat and other gluten-containing substances. (Unfortunately, though, it can take several months to see marked improvement.) The food and substance allergies will be equally difficult to confirm since skin testing can be misleading, and a careful plan of dietary restriction may be the only way to proceed (and this is very difficult for patients to accomplish). Perhaps through negotiation with this patient, with help from a nutritionist, you can establish a basic benign diet that can be added to as tolerated, while other measures are being pursued.

This patient's fixed ideas about "allopathic" medicine will be an obstacle to helping her improve. None of us likes to be in the position to debate our patients. What may work best here is to be supportive of the patient's reasonable skepticism of pharmaceutical therapy—it has not worked for her and has led to side effects—but at the same time to attempt to convince her that the daily acetaminophen–aspirin–caffeine has to be discontinued. It should be done gradually to avoid caffeine withdrawal. A short course of corticosteroid medication can help patients remain comfortable while attempting to discontinue analgesics. It may be possible to convince this patient to go along with a 10-day course of prednisone beginning with 60 mg for 3 or 4 days and then tapering gradually to 0. Magnesium on a daily basis in the 500–600 mg dose range can help chronic migraine and is something she will probably be willing to take. A search for prophylactic and acute medications with little or no coloring may yield some candidates. Several of the cyclic antidepressants and some of the triptans and non-steroidal anti-inflammatory drugs (NSAIDs) fit these requirements, and with the help of a knowledgeable pharmacist, some acceptable options may emerge.

As for nonpharmacological treatment, there is a plethora to choose from and this is the problem. No patient has the time to systematically try all of the "complementary and alternative" options for headaches. Fortunately, there is some evidence for the usefulness of several modalities, including relaxation techniques, cognitive behavioral therapy, and thermal and electromyographic biofeedback (See Table 23–1). Acupuncture, hypnotherapy, and massage therapy have some scientific support. Of the vitamin and herbal therapies, magnesium, coenzyme Q_{10}, riboflavin (vitamin B_2), feverfew (leaf), and butterbur (*Petasites* root) are supported by some evidence. Chiropractic treatment has yet to be shown to be effective for headaches. The so-called energy therapies, including Reiki, craniosacral therapy, qi gong, and meditation, are also proposed widely; but scientific support is not yet available.

There is the possibility that this patient has an anxiety disorder, delusional thought content, or a personality disorder. Anxiety (including generalized anxiety disorder and panic disorder) is comorbid with migraine

TABLE 23-1 **Effective Nonpharmacological, Vitamin, and Herbal Treatments of Migraine and Other Headaches**

Biofeedback–thermal and electromyographic
Cognitive behavioral therapy
Relaxation training
Acupuncture
Magnesium 500-600 mg daily
Vitamin B_2 (riboflavin) 400 mg daily
Coenzyme Q_{10} 200-300 mg daily
Butterbur (petasites) 100-150 mg daily
Feverfew, three capsules of desiccated leaf daily

and can obviously add complexity to the clinician's task. Psychiatric or psychological consultation can help. Delusional or obsessive features are more difficult to assess since they may represent personality style rather than true psychological illness. The presence of a serious thought disorder in this case is very unlikely, unless there is some hidden history. Treatment of anxiety- and personality-driven behavior might well be addressed by a psychologist who has expertise in pain treatment and cognitive behavioral therapy.

> ### KEY POINTS TO REMEMBER
>
> - Over-the-counter medications such as NSAIDs and, in particular, combination medications like acetaminophen-aspirin-caffeine can lead to medication overuse headache, which can mimic primary CDH.
> - Food and other environmental allergies are rarely causes of headaches in the absence of other symptoms.
> - Nonpharmacological therapies which are evidence-based include cognitive behavioral therapy, relaxation techniques, and biofeedback. Biofeedback and massage have some support.
> - Herbal/vitamin headache therapies which have some scientific support include magnesium, vitamin B2, feverfew, butterbur, and coenzyme Q10.

Further Reading

Holroyd KA, Mauskop A. Complementary and alternative treatments. Neurology 2003; 60(suppl):s58-s62.

Limmroth V, Katsarava Z, Fritsche G, Przywara S, Diener HC. Features of medication overuse headache following overuse of different acute headache drugs. Neurology 2002;59(7):1011-1014.

Mathew NT, Kurman R, Perez F. Drug induced refractory headache: clinical features and management. Headache 1990;30:634-638.

Vickers AJ, Rees RW, Zollman CE, et al. Acupuncture for chronic headache in primary care: large, pragmatic, randomised trial. BMJ 2004;328:744-750.

Headache Treatment in Human Immunodeficiency Virus Infection and Drug Addiction

A 48-year-old ex-intravenous drug abuser with human immunodeficiency virus (HIV) but normal white blood cell counts on antiretroviral agents has two to three severe headaches per week which respond to oxycodone prescribed by his former primary-care physician. These headaches have been present "for years," are generally unilateral and throbbing, and can be accompanied by nausea and photophobia. No prophylactic medications have worked, and triptans are contraindicated by the finding of a "silent myocardial infarction" on his electrocardiogram (ECG). Magnetic resonance imaging (MRI) without and with gadolinium done last year was negative. Exam is remarkable only for some stocking pattern sensory loss in the lower extremities.

What do you do now?

This case would challenge a seasoned headache specialist. What often works best in complex headache cases is to break them down into components. Here, the key questions revolve around (*1*) diagnosis, (*2*) choices for acute relief of migraine when triptans are contraindicated, and (*3*) the use of addictive analgesics in patients with a known tendency for drug abuse.

Regarding diagnosis, while migraine is very possible, there are a number of other possibilities. In this case, the MRI speaks against intracranial infection or neoplasm, at least at the time it was done. He presumably has no signs of meningeal irritation, so meningitis as a cause of headaches is unlikely as well. However, a new intracranial mass, infection, hydrocephalus, or arteritis could all be possible, so a repeat MRI (as well as perhaps MR angiography and MR venography) and lumbar puncture would be reasonable in this case. The virus can cause headaches itself, perhaps on the basis of active central nervous system (CNS) infection or due to the fact that the metabolism of serotonin and tryptophan seems to be altered in HIV infection. Antivirals used in HIV-infected patients can lead to headaches as well (and may be the cause of the peripheral neuropathy here). However, Mirsattari et al. (1999) found that primary headaches in patients with HIV infection are very common and usually not related to the antiretroviral drug therapy. They concluded that many cases do not require neuroradiological and/or cerebrospinal fluid examination.

If work-up is unrevealing and exam remains stable, it would seem reasonable to treat this man's headaches as migraine. Prophylactic medication is indicated due to the frequency and the recurring need for analgesia. Beta-blockers, tricyclic antidepressants, topiramate, and perhaps calcium channel blockers might make good choices; but there are risks. Beta-blockers should be used with caution with atazanavir because of the tendency for both to prolong the P–R interval. Ritonavir and other protease inhibitors suppress some hepatic enzyme systems (e.g., cytochrome P-450 3A4 [CYP 3A4]) which could elevate other medication levels (e.g., calcium channel blockers as well as ergots and eletriptan). There is some evidence that valproate may lead to increased replication of HIV. Finally, topiramate induces CYP 3A4 and, thus, can decrease protease inhibitor levels with possible reactivation of the HIV infection.

As for nontriptan acute antimigraine agents, non-steroidal anti-inflammatory drugs, ismetheptene mucate (Midrin), and antinauseant medications such as promethazine (Phenergan) 25 mg po or suppository or metoclopramide (Reglan) 10 mg po might prove effective here. The ECG finding noted above should probably be followed up, possibly with cardiac stress testing and/or catheterization, and a formal decision by an internist or cardiologist about the safety of triptans in this patient. If not contraindicated, triptan treatment might prove highly beneficial.

Opioids have limited use in migraine. While there is some benefit to adding them to other analgesic/abortive agents for particularly severe migraine, regular use of opioids for headaches generally leads to abuse and, at the very least, tolerance and increasing doses. Diverting opioids for the purpose of illicit selling for profit is an increasing problem as well. Despite these drawbacks, opioid use as rescue medication might be reasonable in this case if strict limits on amounts are set and the patient signs an opioid medication contract which includes the agreement to undergo polydrug testing on a regular basis. Other key features of an opioid contract should include provisions to (1) prevent obtaining prescriptions for analgesics from more than one source, (2) ensure compliance with instructions about proper usage of medications, and (3) maintain a schedule of regular office visits. Contracts should also include details about consequences should any part of the agreement not be kept. Opioid contract samples are available at most institutions and on the Internet, including the home sites of the American Pain Society (www.ampainsoc.org), the American Academy for Pain Medicine (www.painmed.org), and the International Association for the Study of Pain (www.iasp-pain.org).

KEY POINTS TO REMEMBER

- There are several ways that HIV can lead to headaches: (1) a direct consequence of the CNS HIV infection (perhaps due to neurotransmitter alteration), (2) opportunistic infections of the head and neck including meningitis and cerebral toxoplasmosis, (3) intracranial neoplasms, and (4) as an adverse effect of antiretroviral or other medications used to treat HIV or HIV-related disease.

Continued

- Opioids are occasionally effective as adjunctive treatment in the setting of acute migraine, but their use as a regular abortive treatment is limited.
- When using opioids or other drugs with addictive potential, strict medication limits, contracts, and drug testing are often indicated.

Further Reading

Arnold RM, Han PK, Seltzer D. Opioid contracts in chronic nonmalignant pain management: objectives and uncertainties. Am J Med 2006;119:292-296.

Coleman I, Rothney A, Wright SC, et al. Use of narcotic analgesics in the emergency department treatment of migraine headache. Neurology 2004;62:1695-1700.

Dodick D, Lipton RB, Martin V, et al. Consensus statement. Cardiovascular safety profile of triptans (5-HT1B/1D agonists) in the acute treatment of migraine. Headache 2004;44:414-425.

Goldstein J. Headache and acquired immunodeficiency syndrome. Neurol Clin 1990;8:947-960.

Mirsattari S, Power C, Nath A. Primary headaches in HIV-infected patients. Headache 1999;39:3-10.

Ziegler DK. Opioids in headache treatment. Is there a role? Neurol Clin 1997;15:199-207.

Pseudotumor

A 24-year-old obese woman began having global
aching and throbbing headaches last year that were
unassociated with nausea, vomiting, or photophobia.
She reports occasional pulsatile tinnitus. Papilledema
was noted after several months and has lessened more
recently. Magnetic resonance imaging (MRI) of the brain
was normal, as were neurological and general exams.
Lumbar puncture (LP) revealed an opening pressure of
28 cm of H_2O. Cerebrospinal fluid (CSF) was acellular and
otherwise normal. She did not notice an improvement
in head pain after LP. A second LP revealed an opening
pressure of 31 cm of H_2O. She is using ibuprofen,
acetaminophen, and hydrocodone nearly daily.
Acetazolamide has caused unpleasant paresthesias in
her hands and feet at the current dose of 200 mg daily;
it does seem to help headaches but not enough.

What do you do now?

P seudotumor cerebri, better termed "idiopathic intracranial hypertension" (IIH), is seen predominantly in obese young women, prompting the concept that venous outflow resistance is causal. However, IIH does occur in nonobese individuals. Some have proposed a pathophysiological dysfunction in the arachnoid granulations as the cause. The presentation is usually fairly pathognomonic—headache, papilledema, and pulsatile tinnitus. Papilledema can be asymmetrical, and some patients do not develop it. Occasionally, some radicular pain in the upper extremities is reported, and some patients experience transient visual obscurations. The LP opening pressure should be above 25 cm. Sixth nerve palsies can occur with symptoms of horizontal diplopia. Visual field testing can reveal an enlarged blind spot. An MRI scan of the head is generally normal, although empty sella, flattening of the globes posteriorly, and small ("slit-like") ventricles have been reported by some authors. Several medications have been implicated in the genesis of intracranial hypertension including vitamin A–related compounds (such as isotretinoin, Accutane), corticosteroids, cimetidine, thyroid medications, estrogenic medications, lithium, and tetracycline.

After MRI rules out mass lesions and hydrocephalus, as it did in this patient, other possibilities include lupus, lupus anticoagulant syndrome, Lyme disease (as well as other chronic meningitides like tuberculosis, syphilis, and *Cryptococcus* infection), cerebral venous thrombosis, leukemia, and migraine. Magnetic resonance venography is indicated in all patients with atypical presentations as a number of patients diagnosed with IIH have later been shown to have occlusion of one or more cerebral veins. (A number of patients with IIH have been found to have significant asymmetry in the size of their transverse venous sinuses, the significance of which is not yet clear.) Thyroid and other hormonal abnormalities have been implicated as well, so thyroid-stimulating hormone, growth hormone, ANA, lupus anticoagulant, anticardiolipin antibody, VDRL, Lyme titer, CBC, and perhaps HIV testing should be done. Pregnancy is said to be a risk factor for the development of IIH, but evidence seems to be lacking. Still, a pregnancy test is worthwhile in all potentially pregnant patients.

In cases like this one, the first step is to make sure the work-up is negative. Next, you need to convince yourself this is really IIH, rather than a primary chronic daily headache. For example, was the LP done in the lateral decubitus position? (If done sitting or even prone, as is typical in fluoroscopically guided LPs, the opening pressure can be falsely elevated.) Migraine features are not present here, but chronic tension-type headache and chronic migraine, perhaps complicated by medication overuse headache, are possibilities. The papilledema and high opening pressures (if accurate) would seem compelling for the diagnosis of IIH in our case, at least for now.

Thus, there are really only two concerns at this point: (1) pain control and (2) prevention of visual compromise, the only actual morbidity encountered in IIH. Monitoring of visual acuity and visual fields by an ophthalmological consultant is therefore essential. Prednisone can reduce CSF pressure and papilledema, in doses of 60–80 mg daily. Long-term treatment is risky, so corticosteroids are usually reserved for exacerbations. If deterioration in vision occurs, optic nerve sheath fenestration (ONF) should be considered. This usually preserves vision; but recurrence of visual impairment can happen later, so this must be followed. Headaches do not generally improve with ONF.

Headache often responds well to acetazolamide, which reduces CSF production via its inhibition of carbonic anhydrase; but some patients find it intolerable. The addition of furosemide may help reduce headaches and might be an option here, which might allow a decrease in acetazolamide. Digoxin supposedly reduces the production of CSF and has been used for some patients effectively. As long as visual acuity is stable, experimenting with medications used for treating primary headaches is reasonable. For example, amitriptyline or nortriptyline, topiramate (which has some carbonic anhydrase inhibiting activity itself, like acetazolamide), other anticonvulsants, and beta-blockers are worth considering. Headaches do not seem to improve after LP, but lumboperitoneal shunting is widely used despite the fact that complications are frequent (e.g., dislodgment or other failure of shunt and infection).

Finally, since obesity clearly impedes venous drainage in the head, weight loss in obese patients like this one is considered a key treatment goal. When patients are unable to accomplish this, gastric bypass is a real consideration, when either headaches or visual effects are intractable.

- Idiopathic intracranial hypertension is most likely to occur in young obese women but can occur in other groups as well.
- Diagnosing IIH is based on elevated CSF pressure as well as the characteristic features of global headache, pulsatile tinnitus, and papilledema.
- Differential diagnosis includes cerebral venous thrombosis, so MRI should also include venography. Lupus and endocrinological disease can lead to increased intracranial pressure, so rheumatological and hormonal work-up is also worthwhile.
- The only morbidity in IIH is preventable visual loss, so close monitoring of visual acuity and visual fields is imperative.

Further Reading

Eggenberger ER, Miller NR, Vitale S. Lumboperitoneal shunt for the treatment of pseudotumor cerebri. Neurology 1996;46:1524–1530.

Farb RI, Vanek I, Scott JN, et al. Idiopathic intracranial hypertension: the prevalence and morphology of sinovenous stenosis. Neurology 2003;60(9):1418–1424.

Friedman DI. Idiopathic intracranial hypertension. Curr Pain Headache Rep 2007;11:62–68.

Nampoory MR, Johny KV, Gupta RK, et al. Treatable intracranial hypertension in patients with lupus nephritis. Lupus 1997;6(7):597–602.

Prognostic, Social, and Legal Issues

26 Migraine Treatment and the Serotonin Syndrome

The pharmacist calls to inform you that he will not dispense the "triptan" prescription you wrote for your patient because she is also on a selective serotonin reuptake inhibitor (SSRI). You explain the reasons for your decision, and he relents. Now the patient is on the phone demanding to know why you are willing to risk her life by combining these drugs.

The pharmacist's concern arose from a Food and Drug Administration (FDA) alert issued in 2006 entitled "Potentially Life-Threatening Serotonin Syndrome with Combined Use of SSRIs or SNRIs with Triptan Medications." The serotonin syndrome (SS) results from the use of individual or a combination of medications that cause an increase in the intrasynaptic levels of serotonin. The medications associated with SS include SSRIs, monoamine oxidase inhibitors (MAOIs), tricyclic antidepressants, weight-loss agents (e.g., sibutramine, Meridia), opioids, antiemetics, certain antibiotics (e.g., linezolid, Zyvox), and herbal products (tryptophan, St. John's wort, ginseng). These agents may induce SS at therapeutic dosages, in overdoses, or following medication withdrawal.

Clinically, the SS ranges from mild symptoms to life-threatening effects. The classic clinical triad of SS includes mental status changes, autonomic dysfunction, and neuromuscular abnormalities. The majority of patients develop symptoms within 6 hours of initiating the medication, changing the dose, or overdosing; 74% become symptomatic within 24 hours. Early in the clinical course of SS, the patient may only complain of tremors, stiffness, or akathisia of the lower extremities and there may be associated sweating and palpitations. In more severe cases, patients may exhibit signs of myoclonus, muscular rigidity, and mental status changes. In its most severe form, SS is associated with hyperpyrexia, muscular rigidity, delirium, seizures, rhabdomyolysis, and renal failure. Because the symptomatology is so diverse and because many clinicians are unaware of the disorder, SS may not be initially recognized, especially in mild cases. Two diagnostic criteria have been developed. The Sternbach criteria mandate that at least three of the following symptoms develop following the recent addition or increase in a known serotonin agent: mental status changes, agitation, myoclonus, hyperreflexia, diaphoresis, shivering, tremor, diarrhea, ataxia/incoordination, or fever. These symptoms must occur in the absence of other potential etiologies and without any recent addition or increase in a neuroleptic agent. In the setting of a serotonergic medication overdose, these criteria have a sensitivity of 75% and are 96% specific in establishing the diagnosis.

What is the risk of SS in the setting of SSRIs, serotonin–norepinephrine reuptake inhibitors (SNRIs), and the triptans? Evans (2007) reviewed the 29 cases upon which the FDA alert was based (27 original reports and two subsequent patients). In his review of the records, obtained through the

Freedom of Information Act, only seven of the cases met the Sternbach criteria. Furthermore, Shapiro and Tepper (2007) estimated that there were nearly 1 million relevant patient–month exposures to triptans and SSRIs during the time in which the FDA made its determination. They extrapolated from these numbers that if only 10% of actual cases were reported, the estimated annual incidence of SS was <0.03% and that the annual incidence of life-threatening SS was <0.002% in patients using both classes of medications. There have not been any reports of triptan monotherapy producing SS, and in a study of more than 1780 patients who were taking both SSRIs and subcutaneous sumatriptan none developed SS.

It is important for the clinician to fully explain the risks and benefits of any medications prior to prescribing them. It is recommended that when triptans are used concurrently with SSRIs or SNRIs the patient is informed of the potential for developing SS, while emphasizing the rarity of the syndrome (<0.03%). The patient should be informed of the characteristic clinical features of SS and instructed to seek treatment urgently should symptoms develop. It is also important for clinicians to be more vigilant in monitoring for signs and symptoms of SS as it has been estimated that approximately 85% of primary-care physicians were unaware of the relationship between antidepressant use and SS. Perhaps the incidence of mild to moderate SS is actually higher but significantly underrecognized and underreported.

KEY POINTS TO REMEMBER

- The SS results from an increase in the concentration of intrasynaptic serotonin.
- The SS may arise from therapeutic doses or overdoses of medications taken alone or in combination and may occasionally follow their withdrawal.
- Implicated medications include MAOIs, SSRIs, SNRIs, tricyclic antidepressants, opioids, antiemetics, and herbal preparations.
- Neuromuscular and autonomic hyperactivity and mental status changes comprise the typical clinical triad.

Continued

- Although an FDA warning was issued regarding the development of the syndrome when SSRIs or SNRIs are combined with triptans, the incidence appears to be very low (<0.03%).
- Clinicians need to be vigilant in monitoring for the condition and to inform their patients of the risks and benefits of combination therapy.

Further Reading

Boyer EW, Shannon M. The serotonin syndrome. N Engl J Med 2005;352:1112–1120.

Evans RW. The FDA alert on serotonin syndrome with combined use of SSRIs or SNRIs and triptans: an analysis of the 29 case reports. Medscape Gen Med 2007;9(3):48.

Mackay FJ, Dunn NR, Mann RD. Antidepressants and the serotonin syndrome in general practice. Br J Gen Pract 1999;49:871–874.

Putnam GP, O'Quinn S, Bolden-Watson CP, et al. Migraine polypharmacy and the tolerability of sumatriptan: a large-scale, prospective study. Cephalalgia 1999;19:668–675.

Shapiro RE, Tepper SJ. The serotonin syndrome, triptans, and the potential for drug–drug interactions. Headache 2007;47:266–269.

Sternbach H. The serotonin syndrome. Am J Psychiatry 1991;148:705–713.

27 School Issues

A 12-year-old boy is in your office for the first time. His parents say he has either left school early or stayed home every day for the past 2 months because of a headache. The history is consistent with a diagnosis of migraine without aura. There is no evidence of comorbid psychological or psychiatric illness. You prescribe acute and preventive treatments and counsel the patient and parents about migraine. As the family is about to leave your office, the parents ask for a note to keep their son out of school until the medications begin to work and add, "What should we do when he says he can't go to school because his headaches are too severe?"

What do you do now?

For the overwhelming majority of children and adolescents with migraine, headache does not result in a significant number of missed days of school. The National Health Interview Survey reported in 2006 that more than 3.7 million children and adolescents aged 4–17 years in the United States had frequent headache pain over a 1-year period. These sufferers with frequent and often intractable headaches account for the majority of missed school days. Clinicians may learn of a patient's excessive school absences in a number of ways: during the course of a routine office visit, during a visit specifically for headache evaluation, from a referral from another physician, through a notification from the school, or as in this case, from a discussion with the parents. However it is discovered, the issue must be dealt with tactfully, professionally, and expediently.

If absences are the result of frequent, disabling headaches, treatment options to lessen headache frequency and severity must be initiated. At times, the clinician may discover that missed school is not the result of acute headache per se but, rather, specific consequences of the chronic illness. Fear of headaches, diminished school performance, lack of sympathy in the classroom, and ridicule by peers may all contribute to the student's reluctance to go to school. Children often mention school as being a headache trigger. Poor school performance in the setting of perceived high expectations (which may be real or imagined) from family members or educators might cause undue stress. This stress may lead to absenteeism directly by triggering headaches or indirectly as a means of avoiding stress. If further probing reveals a pattern of school avoidance (vague symptoms, headaches that occur predominantly during school hours and remit in the evenings and during weekends and vacations), then these issues must be explored and addressed. Nonheadache causes for school avoidance may include bullying or other types of harassment at school, separation anxiety, other home issues (i.e., a perceived need to be at home), learning disabilities, substance abuse, and mental illness.

Parental perceptions may also play a role in keeping the child out of school. In some families, one or both parents may also be migraine sufferers and identify with the child's pain. In these situations, the parents may reinforce the pain behavior; if the child is perceived as "ill," absences may be longer than necessary. Busy work schedules, parental discord, and differences in parenting approaches may all contribute to excessive absenteeism.

In some circumstances, parents and teachers view a child's complaint of headaches and other chronic somatic disorders as a more acceptable reason to miss school than anxiety, depression, or a poor self-image. The management of the child with excessive absenteeism or school avoidance must be tailored to the individual patient. At times, the support and reassurance of the primary health-care provider is all that is needed; in more difficult cases, a multidisciplinary approach involving the student, the parents, and the school system is required. Individual and family counseling are an integral part of the therapeutic regimen and must address the child's coping skills and parental reinforcement of pain behavior. As Lewis and Lake (2001) discuss, behavioral contracts that specify a plan for school attendance with reinforcement contingencies for compliance are particularly useful in this setting. These contracts vary with the individual patient; for some, a gradual return to school, during which the student is expected to attend school for a set number of hours daily regardless of headache intensity, is recommended, while more recalcitrant patients may be required to return to school on a full-time basis. These contracts should stipulate that failure to comply may result in termination of treatment. The clinician must be willing to facilitate the overall care of the patient and collaborate with the other practioners, family members, and school system. The clinician must also set limits, specifying parameters for missing school, documenting dates of absences, and determining the length of the absences. School personnel should be educated about the condition and its impact upon the sufferer, to avoid further stigmatizing the child. Medication issues should be reviewed with the school nurse so that acute therapy is not delayed and a quiet room is provided if needed.

In summary, an optimal scenario in this case might proceed as follows. Our patient and his parents were referred to a psychologist for individual and family therapy. A behavioral contract was drawn up in which the patient agreed (reluctantly) to return to school full-time as a condition of his treatment. The parents were educated regarding the importance of school attendance and the implications of excessive absenteeism. They were counseled individually and together with their son, with specific recommendations as to how to deal with their child's headaches. Positive reinforcement models were outlined and strategies to avoid negative reinforcement patterns suggested.

- School issues should be routinely addressed during consultations with children, adolescents, and their parents.
- Frequent intractable headaches or fear of headaches, diminished school performance, lack of sympathy in the classroom, and ridicule by peers may all contribute to the student's reluctance to go to school.
- Nonheadache issues may underlie school avoidance and must be searched for.
- Treatment should involve the patient, parents, and school personnel.
- Consider the use of behavioral contracts as well as individual and family psychotherapy.
- Returning to school is the goal, with consideration of homebound programs only as a last resort.

Further Reading

Green M. The "vulnerable child": intimations of mortality. Pediatrics 1980;65:1042-1043.

Lewis DW, Lake AE. Psychologic and nonpharmacologic treatment of headache. In: Winner P, Rothner DA (eds), Headache in Children and Adolescents. New York: BC Decker, 2001, pp 126-141.

Lewis DW, Middlebrook MT, Mehallick L, et al. Pediatric headache: what do the children want? Headache 1996;36:224-230.

Smith MS. Psychosomatic symptoms in adolescents. Med Clin North Am 1990;74:1121-1134.

Stang PE, Osterhouse JT. Impact of migraine in the United States: data from the National Health Interview Survey. Headache 1993;33:29-35.

US Department of Health and Human Services, Centers for Disease Control and Prevention. 2006 National Health Interview Survey (NHIS) Public Use Data Release. Hyattsville, MD: 2006.

Wall BA, Holden EW, Gladstone J. Parent responses to pediatric headache. Headache 1997;37:65-70.

Posttraumatic Headaches

A 46-year-old woman describes severe global headaches
since a motor vehicle accident 1 year ago. She does
not remember whether or not she struck her head and
thinks that she did not lose consciousness. She did not
seek medical help immediately. Neck and midback pain
began the day after the accident and resolved in several
days. Headaches began approximately 2 weeks after the
accident and have persisted. The headaches are nearly
daily, nonnauseating, and accompanied by fatigue and
malaise. The patient also complains of poor concentration
and intermittent dizziness since her accident. The
headaches and her other symptoms have led to the loss
of her job (one she very much valued) and to marital
discord. The other vehicle in the accident was found to
be "at fault." Cervical spine magnetic resonance imaging
(MRI) reveals "straightening" and mild midcervical
arthritic changes. There is an ongoing lawsuit claiming
that permanent damage was done and asking for a
multimillion-dollar payment. The patient wants you to
diagnose traumatic causation and to testify to this effect.

What do you do now?

ecoming enmeshed in the legal dealings of patients is something most physicians will work very hard to avoid. Unfortunately, it sometimes goes with the territory when working with headache and pain patients. The best first steps are, as usual, to formulate the proper diagnosis or diagnoses, decide on therapeutic goals with the patient, and think about the best routes for reaching these goals. Putting the legal considerations into a separate category seems to work best since the type of thinking and documentation can be very different from medical models.

In this case a posttraumatic syndrome seems likely, unless the patient is malingering. While the latter is possible, it seems unlikely given the highly negative impact her illness has had on her life (no guarantee of course). The *International Classification of Headache Disorders*, second edition (ICHD-II) defines both posttraumatic headaches and postwhiplash headaches (see Tables 28–1 and 28–2), which can become chronic as in this case. However, both diagnoses rest on the appearance of headaches within 7 days following the injury, not true in the case above. There is really no clear understanding of how head and neck trauma causes persistent headaches. Likewise, there are really no tests to determine whether an actual injury was done in most cases. Nonetheless, there is significant clinical support for the existence of posttraumatic headaches, sometimes lasting for years, following head trauma (even mild as in this case) or "whiplash" injury.

TABLE 28-1   ICHD Chronic Posttraumatic Headache Attributed to Mild Head Injury

Diagnostic criteria

A. Headache, no typical characteristics known, fulfilling criteria C and D

B. Head trauma with all of the following:
   1. Either no loss of consciousness or loss of consciousness of <30 minutes' duration
   2. Glasgow Coma Scale >13
   3. Symptoms and/or signs diagnostic of concussion

C. Headache develops within 7 days after head trauma

D. Headache persists for >3 months after head trauma

TABLE 28-2 ICHD-II Chronic Headache Attributed to Whiplash Injury

Diagnostic criteria

A. Headache, no typical characteristics known, fulfilling criteria C and D

B. History of whiplash (sudden and significant acceleration/deceleration movement of the neck) associated at the time with neck pain

C. Headache develops within 7 days after whiplash injury

D. Headache persists for >3 months after whiplash injury

TABLE 28-3 Symptoms of the Postconcussive Syndrome

- Headaches
- Dizziness, light-headedness, vertigo
- Visual blurring
- Hearing loss and/or tinnitus
- Fatigue
- Irritability, mood disturbance, anxiety
- Memory, concentration, or other cognitive impairment
- Sleep dysfunction
- Sexual dysfunction

As for this patient's other symptoms—fatigue, malaise during the headaches, and poor concentration and intermittent dizziness at other times—these would seem to imply a "postconcussion syndrome" (PCS), defined by the psychiatric *Diagnostic and Statistical Manual* (DSM-IV) as "postconcussional disorder." This controversial disorder can be characterized by a myriad of symptoms (see Table 28–3), the most common of which is headache. The pathophysiology of this condition too is unknown, although diffuse axonal injury due to acceleration/deceleration forces has been postulated, with most severe effects thought to be present frontotemporally, based on known results of head trauma and autopsy studies.

Many patients with chronic posttraumatic headaches are given psychological diagnoses or are considered drug-seeking or malingerers. However, the commonly held belief that a large money settlement will "cure" the syndrome has been shown to be spurious (see Packard, 1992). Supporting this patient's legal claim will still be challenging. First, there is likely to be no evidence for brain injury. An MRI of the head can sometimes reveal areas of encephalomalacia or leukomalacia consistent with traumatic brain contusion or other damage sustained at the time of injury. Neuropsychiatric testing can be supportive as well, if there are findings of PCS-type cognitive compromise and low malingering scores. A delay in the late cerebral evoked potential P300 can be supportive as well, but this is controversial. Electroencephalography is generally unhelpful unless a seizure focus is found, but functional central nervous system imaging has the potential in the future to be of help. In fact, positron emission tomographic scan abnormalities have been used in legal arguments regarding posttraumatic syndromes.

Another tricky issue is the timing of this patient's headache onset—1 week later than the ICHD definitions require. Not an obstacle to the appropriate clinical impression, but one could imagine the opposing attorney brandishing a copy of the ICHD-II and asking whether or not it is the accepted source for defining headaches. On clinical grounds, however, a physician confidently stating a diagnosis can be very compelling. Whether or not to embark on this path is up to the individual physician, but it is important to remember that you may be your patient's only advocate here. To promote clarity, it is best to be decisive in documenting your clinical impressions. The legal world tends to disregard the common medical approach of "possible" or "rule-out" diagnoses. So, a reasonable statement in a medical note impression on the above case might be "This patient has a posttraumatic headache disorder, more likely than not due to the motor vehicle accident described above." To avoid unmanageable time commitments, many of us find it useful to be available (for a reasonable fee and at specific times) to provide testimony at a deposition but not to make court appearances. It is very rare that a court will not recognize the time constraints of physicians.

As for treatment, despite the lack of good evidence for pharmacological and nonpharmacological options, many patients have been helped by a combination of lifestyle, cognitive behavioral, and pharmacological therapies. A good place to begin is to make a thorough search for treatable causes of pain such as occipital or supraorbital neuritis, cervical spine pathology, and musculoskeletal dysfunction of other types. (Persistent cerebrospinal fluid leak, traumatic vascular malformations, and cerebral venous thrombosis, while unlikely in the chronic form or posttraumatic headaches, should also be kept in mind.) Posttraumatic headaches can take many forms including migraine, tension-type headache, and even cluster headache. What seems to work best in terms of medication choices are those agents best suited for the headache presentation, both prophylactically and for the acute relief of breakthrough severe headaches. Here, where there are few migraine features, a chronic daily headache prophylactic agent such as a tricyclic antidepressant or an anticonvulsant medication might be effective along with lifestyle changes and other approaches discussed in previous chapter. Non-steroidal anti-inflammatory drugs or possibly triptan medication could be effective acutely.

KEY POINTS TO REMEMBER

- Mild head and/or neck trauma can lead to chronic headaches, although the specific mechanisms are not clear.
- The headache disorder may be a component of the postconcussive syndrome.
- Associated injuries to superficial nerves and the cervical spine can be the cause of posttraumatic headaches.
- The ICHD-II definition of posttraumatic headache requires the onset of head pain within a week of the injury, but there are exceptions in clinical practice.

Further Reading

American Psychiatric Association. Diagnostic and Statistical Manual of Mental Disorders, DSM-IV-TR, 4th ed, text rev. Washington DC: American Psychiatric Association, 2000.

Packard RC. Posttraumatic headache permanency and relationship to legal settlement. Headache 1992;32:496–500.

Solomon S. Posttraumatic headache. Med Clin North Am 2001;85(4):987–996.

Weeks R. Post-traumatic headache. In: Levin M, Ward TN (eds), Head, Neck and Facial Pain. Columbus, OH: Anadem, 2006.

Young WB, Packard RC, Katsarava Z. Headaches associated with head trauma. In: Wolff's headache and other head pain. New York: Oxford University Press, 2008.

29 Transient Global Amnesia and Migraine

A 50-year-old man with a history of migraine with aura returns for a follow-up visit after a 2-year absence. In reviewing his medical history, he reveals that he had an episode of transient global amnesia (TGA) last year with a negative work-up that included magnetic resonance imaging (MRI) of the brain, electroencephalogram, and echocardiogram. His local neurologist has continued to prescribe a "triptan" for his acute attacks, and the patient now requests a refill from you.

What do you do now?

Transient global amnesia is a well-recognized neurological syndrome resulting in a short-lasting inability to create new memory. The disorder occurs more commonly after age 50, with an annual incidence of 23.5 cases per 100,000. Clinically, TGA is characterized by the sudden onset of antero-grade amnesia, during which there is an inability to retain new information without impairment in immediate recall or remote memory. The defect in memory typically resolves within 8–24 hours, leaving the patient with a per-manent amnestic period for the attack duration. The event may be triggered by stressful situations, exertion, immersion in cold water, sexual intercourse, or a minor medical procedure such as endoscopy or angiogram.

The pathophysiology of TGA is unknown. Putative etiologies have included migraine, seizure disorders, and transient ischemic attacks (TIAs); but for the majority of cases, no obvious source is ever identified. In gen-eral, most studies suggest that TIA is not a likely explanation for these events. Patients with TGA have been reported to have fewer cerebrovas-cular risk factors than patients with documented cerebrovascular disease, and except in rare instances, TGA is a one time–only event. However, pos-itron emission tomographic (PET) scans and diffusion-weighted imaging (DWI) studies have demonstrated transient disruption of blood flow to the thalamus, amygdala, and hippocampus during acute episodes of TGA; and a study using single-photon emission computed tomography (SPECT) documented persistent temporal hypoperfusion 3 months after an episode of TGA. Focal hypoperfusion has also been reported to persist in patients with recurrent TGA as long as a year following the event.

Although TGA occurs with an increased frequency in patients with pre-existing migraine, the relationship is weak at best. Most TGA sufferers deny headache or associated nausea, photophobia, or phonophobia during the attack. Interestingly, however, PET, DWI, and SPECT studies performed dur-ing TGA have documented changes consistent with spreading depression.

Recent work suggests that TGA may have a venous rather than an arterial etiology and that there may be two subtypes. In "pure" TGA, in which the sufferer experiences only one attack, internal jugular valvular insufficiency permits the increased venous pressure that occurs during Valsalva maneu-vers to cause venous congestion, which leads to transient ischemia of the mesial temporal structures (amygdala and hippocampus). Recurrent TGA, the second subgroup, may occur in patients with arterial risk factors.

Using triptans in migraine sufferers who had TGA is a cause of debate among headache specialists. Many feel that since TGA is not a TIA and because TGA sufferers have fewer stroke risk factors than patients with TIA, the use of triptans is safe. Furthermore, the notion that TGA may be caused by spreading depression, the same phenomenon believed to be responsible for migraine aura, the use of triptans should not be prohibited. Others believe that TGA may be representative of a transient cerebrovascular event and, therefore, would not allow these patients to continue using triptans. Perhaps, then, a more prudent approach would be to get a DWI, SPECT, or PET scan at the onset of the TGA and to repeat it 24 hours after the event resolves. If these tests are normal, then the triptan may be considered. Abnormalities in the scans or recurrent episodes of TGA would prohibit their use.

KEY POINTS TO REMEMBER

- Transient global amnesia is characterized by the sudden onset of anterograde amnesia without impairment in immediate recall or remote memory.
- Transient global amnesia occurs more commonly after age 50.
- The pathophysiology of TGA is unknown, but it has been postulated to be related to migraine, TIA, or seizure.
- Transient global amnesia may have a venous rather than an arterial etiology.
- The use of triptans in patients with prior TGA is probably safe if work-up is negative and there are no recurrences.

Further Reading

Eustache F, Desgranges B, Petit-Taboué MC, et al. Transient global amnesia: implicit/explicit memory dissociation and PET assessment of brain perfusion and oxygen metabolism in the acute stage. J Neurol Neurosurg Psychiatry 1997;63:357-367.

Lewis SL. Aetiology of transient global amnesia. Lancet 1998;352:397-300.

Menendez Gonzalez M, Martinez Rivera M. Transient global amnesia. Increasing evidence of a venous etiology. Arch Neurol 2006;63:1334-1336.

Pantoni L, Bertini E, Lamassa M, et al. Clinical features, risk factors, and prognosis in transient global amnesia; a follow-up study. Eur J Neurol 2005;12:350-356.

Strupp M, Bruning R, Wu RH, et al. Diffusion-weighted MRI in transient global amnesia: elevated signal intensity in the left mesial temporal lobe in 7 of 10 patients. Ann Neurol 1998;43:164–170.

Winbeck K, Etgen T, von Einsiedel HG, et al. DWI in transient global amnesia and TIA: proposal for an ischaemic origin of TGA. J Neurol Neurosurg Psychiatry 2005;76:438–441.

You are evaluating a 28-year-old man with a 5-year history of predominantly right-sided headaches that are typical of migraine without aura. He is otherwise healthy. Family history is remarkable for an uncle who died of a brain hemorrhage. Since his headaches have never occurred on the opposite side, you order magnetic resonance imaging (MRI) of the brain, despite his normal exam. The MRI reveals a left-sided arteriovenous malformation (AVM) (Fig. 30-1).

What do you do now?

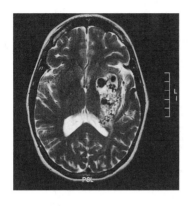

FIGURE 30-1 Arteriovenous malformation. (Courtesy of Gordon Heller, MD, Department of Neuro-Radiology, Roosevelt Hospital Center, New York, NY.)

Arteriovenous malformations are congenital lesions that are composed of tangles of arteries and veins that form a fistula. These supratentorial lesions have no capillary bed, which allows the feeding arteries to empty directly into the draining veins. The exact prevalence of cerebral AVMs is not known but is estimated to be approximately 0.1%. Although the majority of patients with AVMs come to medical attention only after they are symptomatic, the widespread availability of MRI has significantly increased the numbers of patients found incidentally to harbor unruptured AVMs.

Clinically, cerebral AVMs may present as hemorrhages (intracerebral, subarachnoid, or intraventricular), seizures (focal or generalized), headaches, focal neurological deficits, and pulsatile tinnitus. Approximately 14% of patients with known AVMs report chronic headaches, unrelated to hemorrhage. These headaches may have features of migraine and are usually ipsilateral to the lesion. Migraine with aura has been reported in 58% of women with AVMs. These vascular abnormalities have also been reported in association with atypical presentations of cluster, chronic paroxysmal hemicrania (CPH), and the SUNCT (short-lasting, unilateral, neuralgiform headache attacks with conjunctival injection and tearing) syndrome.

Our patient has typical migraine without aura that, when unilateral, is always right-sided. His AVM is on the asymptomatic side and is most likely an incidental finding and not causative. Although we can reasonably say that the lesion is not responsible for this patient's headache, is any further work-up necessary, and does the AVM warrant treatment?

The most worrisome feature of an AVM is its potential to hemorrhage; bleeding is associated with a mortality rate of 10%–30% and a morbidity rate of 20%–30%. The long-term risk for hemorrhage is approximately 1%–3% yearly, and this risk is elevated in patients who have presented with bleeds. The risk of recurrent hemorrhage in the first year is 6%–17% and rises to approximately 25% in the first year for patients who have had a second bleed. The rate of bleeding in unruptured AVMs also varies with the vascular anatomy and location of the lesion. A deep brain location and the presence of deep venous drainage increase the likelihood of a first bleed.

The lifetime risk of bleeding from an unruptured AVM can be estimated by using the following formula: Lifetime risk (%) = 105 – patient's age in years (Brown et al, 2005). This suggests that our patient has a 77% chance of bleeding over the course of his life, yet how he should be treated is not clear. Recent prospective data suggest that interventional therapy is associated with a very highly significant increased risk of subsequent bleeding and disability when compared with conservative management. In this study of 352 AVM patients, there was a greater than threefold increase in the risk for AVM hemorrhage if patients underwent interventional treatment, which would suggest that conservative management should be very strongly considered (Staph et al, 2006). However, others argue that our patient has a life expectancy of an additional 50 years, and the risk of bleeding during this time is too high to do nothing (Cockroft, 2007). Unfortunately, we are still left with the dilemma of which interventional therapy to recommend (microsurgical, radiosurgical, or embolization) as none has been evaluated in controlled trials. A randomized study of adults over age 18 with unruptured brain AVMs will attempt to answer the question of whether conservative management is superior to any of the interventional approaches (see ARUBA study). Until this study is completed, the decision of how to treat should incorporate a multidisciplinary approach involving the neurologist, neurosurgeon, neuroradiologist, and interventional neuroradiologist. Treatment decisions must weigh the potential for benefit against the potential risk of both the natural history of the disorder (morbidity and mortality) and the therapeutic intervention.

Further Reading

Brown RD, Flemming KD, Meyer FB, et al. Natural history, evaluation, and management of intracranial vascular malformations. Mayo Clin Proc 2005;80:269-281.

Cockroft K. Unruptured brain arteriovenous malformations should be treated conservatively: no. Stroke. 2007;38:3310-3311

Hofmeister C, Stapf C, Hartmann A, et al. Demographic, morphological, and clinical characteristics of 1289 patients with brain arteriovenous malformations. Stroke 2000;31:1307-1310.

Randomized Multicenter Clinical Trial of Unruptured Brain AVMs (ARUBA). http://www.arubastudy.org/frameSetDescripTrial.html

Stapf C, Mohr JP, Choi JH, et al. Invasive treatment of unruptured brain arteriovenous malformations is experimental therapy. Curr Opin Neurol 2006;19:63-68.

31 Migraine and Patent Foramen Ovale

A longtime patient of yours with migraine with aura, well controlled with acute treatment (naratriptan), recently learned about the alleged link between migraine and "holes in the heart." She had one episode of transient mental status change last year, which led to an emergency room visit, diagnosis of transient ischemic attack (TIA), and negative work-up including computed tomography of the head that night. Electroencephalogram, echocardiogram, and magnetic resonance imaging (including diffusion weight mode) were all normal the next day. She wants to have you investigate further to see if she has a patent foramen ovale (PFO) and arrange for its repair if found. She is 56, on no daily medications, and otherwise healthy. Her general and neurological exams are normal.

What do you do now?

This patient's interest in the PFO "story" is not unusual. The facts have been sensationalized, and many have heard about the possibility of a migraine "cure" when PFO repair is done. Here are some key facts:

1. Around 25% of people have PFO.
2. Around 50% of migraine sufferers have PFO.
3. People with migraine with aura have a much higher risk of having a large PFO than the general population.
4. A number of open-label studies have shown very significant improvement in migraine frequency in patients with migraine with aura after percutaneous PFO closure.

However, like so much data in medical research, interpretation and application to one's own patients can be nearly impossible. Yes, many migraine sufferers have PFO, but it is important to remember that most are potential defects only, with no right to left shunting of blood in any situation. The observation of a five- to sixfold increased risk of having a "significant" PFO in patients with migraine with aura is much more compelling for the presence of a link between PFO and migraine with aura. On the other hand, the definition of "significant" can vary—whether based on size (determined by a probe versus appearance on echocardiogram) or degree of shunting of blood (which can be subjective when using the echocardiographic bubble technique) (see Fig. 31–1). Studies of PFO in scuba divers by Wilmshurst and colleagues (2000) revealed that individuals with PFO and large right to left shunts have a high incidence of migraine after dives and a very high

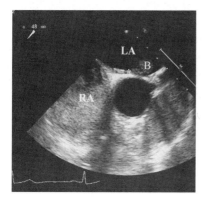

FIGURE 31-1 Echocardiogram image during Valsalva using the "bubble technique" (intravenous injection of agitated saline). Note bubbles (B) present in the left atrium (LA) distal to the PFO (*). RA, right atrium. (Courtesy of Timothy G. Lukovits, MD, Section of Neurology, Dartmouth Hitchcock Medical Center, Lebanon, NH.)

prevalence of migraine at other times (47%). This too seems to link migraine and PFO. But could migraine and PFO be genetically linked with no real medical bearing on each other? An interesting study done by Wilmshurst et al. (2004) concluded that there seems to be an element of dominant inheritance of atrial shunts, which seems to be linked to inheritance of migraine with aura in some families.

How PFOs might predispose to migraine has been food for thought for a number of authors. Some postulated that small emboli or showers of emboli from venous sources cross directly into the left atrium and then to the brain, producing cerebral changes that lead to a migraine. (They could also lead to white matter changes seen in migraineurs, as mentioned later.) Others suggest that certain metabolic products (e.g., nitric oxide or serotonin), normally detoxified in the lungs, pass directly into the cerebral circulation via the PFO, leading again to some physiological state that then lowers the threshold for migraine.

All of these data and conjectures aside, is closure of PFO shunt beneficial to migraine patients? It seems that the new devices using "umbrella"-type deployment via catheter insertion through the femoral vein are relatively safe. There are occasional complications, such as embolization from the apparatus and dislodgement of the closure device, which are daunting but fortunately rare. Yes, a number of open-label studies of transcatheter PFO closure in migraine patients have suggested dramatically beneficial effects on headaches. However, a controlled blinded study done in the United Kingdom in an attempt to prove benefit to migraine sufferers (the Migraine Intervention with STARflex Technology [MIST] study) (Dowson et al. 2008) really showed no benefit over prophylactic medical therapy of migraine. (About 42% of the patients undergoing PFO closure had at least a 50% improvement in migraine frequency compared to 23% who had the "sham" procedure.)

As for the best approach to treating patients who have had TIA or stroke and who have a PFO (regardless of their migraine history), there are as yet no published randomized controlled studies on PFO closure plus medical treatment versus medical treatment alone for the prevention of recurrence of cryptogenic stroke. There are several studies under way, and this will become clearer soon (hopefully). However, did this patient even have a stroke or TIA? It is generally felt that with a negative work-up, as this patient had, and no clear history or examination findings consistent with cerebral ischemia, diagnosing TIA is unreliable.

When patients ask about the stroke risk in migraine, there is actually enough data to draw some conclusions. The increased risk for stroke in migraineurs, around twice normal, is highest for women under age 45 and for patients with migraine and aura. Several studies, particularly the much discussed Kruit et al. (2004) study, show that migraine patients, especially those with long-standing disease and frequent headaches, have a higher risk for cerebral and especially cerebellar white matter lesions. Some patients are aware of this and ask for advice about how to minimize their risks. The problem here is that these lesions are not clearly of any clinical significance, and we do not even know if they are ischemic lesions.

What most headache specialists tell patients who are concerned about the presence of a PFO is that unless there are symptoms other than migraine (hypoxemia, clear previous history of paradoxical embolism, scuba diving complications), closure is not really indicated. Therefore, a search for a "surgical" PFO is not worthwhile. When asked about the risk of stroke in migraine and how to manage it, the best response is to control more significant risks—hypertension, tobacco use, exogenous estrogen use, hyperlipidemia, etc. These would be reasonable approaches in the above patient. The one episode of altered mental state could have been the result of any number of possible causes, including metabolic compromise, medication effects, systemic infection, epilepsy, transient global amnesia, or anxiety. She should be encouraged to report any future similar occurrences without delay.

KEY POINTS TO REMEMBER

- Patent foramen ovale is a common congenital defect which is usually harmless.
- Patients with migraine and aura seem to have a significantly increased risk of larger PFO, which may represent a mechanistic or genetic link.
- There is no clear evidence yet for PFO closure leading to beneficial effects on migraine.

Further Reading

Etminan M, Takkouche B, Isorna F, Samii A. Risk of ischaemic stroke in people with migraine: systematic review and meta-analysis of observational studies. BMJ 2005;330:63–65.

Kruit MC, van Buchem MA, Hofman PA, Bakkers JT, Terwindt GM, Ferrari MD, Launer LJ. Migraine as a risk factor for subclinical brain lesions. JAMA 2004;291:427–434.

Wilmshurst PT, Nightingale S, Walsh KP, Morrison WL. Effect on migraine closure of cardiac right-to-left shunts to prevent recurrence of decompression illness or stroke or for haemodynamic reasons. Lancet 2000;356:1648–1651.

Wilmshurst PT, Pearson MJ, Nightingale S, Walsh KP, Morrison WL. Inheritance of persistent foramen ovale and atrial septal defects and the relation to familial migraine with aura. Heart 2004;90:1315–1320.Dowson A, Mullen MJ, Peatfield R, et al. A prospective, multicenter, double-blind, sham-controlled trial to evaluate the effectiveness of patent foramen ovale closure with starflex septal repair implant to resolve refractory migraine headache. Circulation 2008;117:1397–1404

32 Postconcussive Headache

A 15-year-old boy is brought in by his father. The child is the starting quarterback on the high school varsity squad. Last week he suffered a "mild" concussion, which caused some transient memory loss and altered behavior; but he returned to normal over the next 2 days. There was no apparent loss of consciousness. His coach says he is fine now and wants him to be the starting quarterback in the playoff game this weekend (in 3 days) but requires a note from you clearing him to play. His exam is normal, but he is complaining of a mild, persistent global headache.

What do you do now?

In the United States there are approximately 300,000 sports-related concussions each year; more than 60,000 occur in high school athletes. The majority of the concussions in high school are the result of a football injury. Determining when to allow an athlete to return to competition following a concussion can be a challenging clinical decision, especially because the current guidelines are consensus-, rather than evidence-, based. Further complicating the issue is that concussions are often underreported and their seriousness unrecognized. In the macho world of competitive football, returning to play after getting "dinged" or having one's "bell rung" is considered a sign of toughness, rather than a warning of a concussive brain injury.

The Quality Standard Committee (QSC) of the American Academy of Neurology developed practice parameters for the management of concussion in sports in 1997. These guidelines define *concussion* as a trauma-induced alteration in mental status that may or may not involve loss of consciousness. The document reviews the most common features of concussion, which include a vacant stare or befuddled look, slowed verbal and motor responses, confusion, distractibility, disorientation, dysarthric or incoherent speech, incoordination, emotional lability, memory disturbances, and impairments of consciousness. Postconcussive symptoms may appear soon after the injury (early) and may persist for days to weeks or longer (late). The early symptoms include headache, dizziness, inattention, nausea, and vomiting. Late symptoms can include a continuous low-grade headache, light-headedness, memory impairment, fatigue and distractibility, heightened sensation to lights and sounds, tinnitus, mood and sleep disturbances, and irritability. The pathophysiology underlying acute and late postconcussion syndrome symptoms is still unclear, with lingering beliefs by many in psychological factors. However, S-100 protein and neuron-specific enolase, suggesting neuronal injury, are elevated in many patients; and it is clear in some cases that diffuse axonal injury has occurred.

Concussions are graded by their level of severity. As defined by the QSC, grade 1, the most common, is characterized by transient confusion without a loss of consciousness and with concussive symptoms or mental status abnormalities that resolve in less than 15 minutes. In a grade 2 concussion, the symptoms and mental status abnormalities persist for longer than 15 minutes. The hallmark of a grade 3 concussion is loss of consciousness.

Glasgow Coma Scale grade in concussion is almost always normal or 14/15, so its usefulness is limited.

The QSC has published recommendations delineating when to allow an athlete to return to play following a single event as well as following multiple concussive injuries. For all grades, the athlete should be immediately removed from the contest for evaluation. Grade 1 sufferers may return to the game if mental status abnormalities or postconcussive symptoms completely resolve within 15 minutes; sufferers of grade 2 or grade 3 concussions may not return on the same day. Following a grade 2 concussion, the athlete should be reexamined frequently that day and again the following day. If the neurological examination is normal, the patient may be cleared to return to play as long as he or she remains asymptomatic for a week (both at rest and during exertion). If headaches or other symptoms persist or worsen for longer than 1 week, the QSC recommends neuroimaging. Athletes suffering a grade 3 concussion must be transported to the nearest emergency department for evaluation. They must be neurologically normal and asymptomatic for 1–2 weeks (depending on the length of unconsciousness) before being allowed to return to competition. Recent work with functional magnetic resonance imaging (fMRI) has documented changes in brain function that occur as a result of a concussive injury in high school athletes. In a small study of 28 patients and 13 age-matched controls, fMRIs were obtained within 1 week of a concussion and then again after the subjects improved so that they were cleared to return to play based on current guidelines. The athletes who had abnormal brain activation on the first scan required almost twice as long to recover when compared to those athletes whose initial scans were normal. Functional MRI is not currently employed as part of the postconcussive evaluation; however, its use in the future may help validate existing guidelines so that they are evidence-based.

The adolescent you are currently evaluating meets criteria for a grade 2 concussion. His transient memory loss and behavioral abnormalities lasted longer than 15 minutes before totally resolving. The QSC guidelines recommend that athletes with a grade 2 concussion not be allowed to return to play until they are neurologically cleared (which he is) and asymptomatic for 1 week (which he is not). This boy continues to complain of a mild headache and, therefore, may not be cleared to return to the game.

Furthermore, if his headache persists or worsens for a week or more, an MRI of the brain should be ordered.

How would the situation change if this was not his first concussion? The QSC has also developed guidelines for return to play following multiple concussions. These guidelines suggest that, for multiple grade 1 concussions, the athlete must be neurologically normal and asymptomatic at rest and with exertion for 1 week before being cleared; however, if the second grade 1 concussion occurred on the same day, the player should be removed from the game that day. Multiple grade 2 concussions require 2 weeks, and following multiple grade 3 concussions, a period of 1 month or longer is recommended before the athlete may return to the game. Of course, any abnormality on neuroimaging that is consistent with intracranial pathology (such as cerebral contusions) necessitates termination of that season; if these abnormalities follow a grade 3 concussion, withdrawal from future participation in the sport should be advised.

KEY POINTS TO REMEMBER

- Remove from game for evaluation.
- Grade 1: May return to game the same day if symptoms resolve in less than 15 minutes.
- Grade 2: May not return the same day.
- If neurologically cleared and asymptomatic (at both rest and exertion), may return in 1 week.
- If headache or other symptom persists, neuroimaging is recommended.
- Grade 3: May not return the same day.
- Transport to nearest emergency department.
- If neurologically cleared and asymptomatic (at both rest and exertion), may return in 1 week—if loss of consciousness was brief (seconds).
- If neurologically cleared and asymptomatic (at both rest and exertion), may return in 2 weeks—if loss of consciousness was prolonged (minutes).

Further Reading

Guskiewicz KM, Bruce SL, Cantu RC, et al. Recommendations on management of sport-related concussion: summary of the National Athletic Trainers' Association position statement. Neurosurgery 2004;55:891–896.

Kelly JP, Rosenberg JH. The diagnosis and management of concussion in sports. Neurology 1997;48:575–580.

Lovell MR, Pardini JE, Welling J, et al. Functional brain abnormalities are related to clinical recovery and time to return-to-play in athletes. Neurosurgery 2007;61(2): 352–360.

Powell JW, Barber-Foss KD. Traumatic brain injury in high school athletes. JAMA 1999; 282:958–963.

Quality Standards Subcommittee of the American Academy of Neurology. Practice parameter: the management of concussion in sports (summary statement). Neurology 1997;48:581–585.

33 Use of Triptans in Elderly Patients

A 72-year-old woman with long-standing migraine headaches who you are seeing for the first time reports that her headaches are well-controlled with preventive agents nortriptyline and atenolol. She successfully treats acute attacks with a "triptan" that she uses approximately twice weekly. She has no other medical illnesses other than mild hypercholesterolemia [total cholesterol 230 mg/dl, high-density lipoprotein (HDL) 70 mg/dl] that is well-controlled with simvastatin. She requests refills of all her medications.

What do you do now?

n the United States, people over 65 years of age comprise the fastest-growing segment of the population. Migraine is typically thought of as a disease of young people, and although it is true that migraine rarely has its onset after age 50 and that many migraine sufferers report that their headaches disappear as they get older, the prevalence of migraine in the elderly is significant. Estimates suggest that 3%–10% of the elderly suffer from migraine. These sufferers continue to report migraine-related disability and require treatment.

The use of triptans in the elderly raises several important clinical issues. Some clinicians have an arbitrary age limit above which they do not prescribe these medications; others will use these agents as long as there are no medical contraindications. Given that these agents were not tested in the elderly, the increased risk of medical comorbidities (especially cardiac and cerebrovascular diseases) and polypharmacy that occurs in older patients, as well as the changes in drug metabolism and elimination that may occur as patients age, the decision-making process here is difficult. Many patients who began using these medications decades ago have now reached the age at which their heath-care providers are uncomfortable with or unwilling to continue prescribing. In the absence of formal guidelines, how do we decide?

The package inserts for all the triptans state that these medications are contraindicated for patients with risk factors for coronary artery disease (CAD) unless they have undergone a "thorough cardiovascular evaluation" which provides "satisfactory clinical evidence" that cardiovascular disease has been excluded. These package inserts do not specify what this evaluation should include. Some clinicians interpret this to mean that all patients who are at risk for cardiac disease be screened with electrocardiography (EKG) and stress tests prior to being prescribed triptans. Yet, the limitations of these tests to document asymptomatic CAD are well described, and in fact those same package inserts state "the sensitivity of cardiac diagnostic procedures to detect cardiovascular disease or predisposition to coronary artery vasospasm is modest, at best." Because of these limitations, some have proposed that this cardiac evaluation consist of risk factor stratification based on results from the Framingham Study. This model incorporates six variables (gender, total cholesterol levels, HDL levels, blood pressure, presence or absence of diabetes, and tobacco use) and is capable of providing reliable 10-year estimates of a patient's CAD risk. This method allows patients to be stratified into low (<10% risk of symptomatic CAD within the next 10 years), intermediate (>10% but <20%), or high (>20%) risk groups. Patients often report that their migraines become less severe with advancing age. For these patients, a trial of a previously ineffective symptomatic medication may be warranted. Remember, however, that non-steroidal anti-inflammatory drugs and aspirin may also be more likely to induce bleeding in the elderly and may interact with other medications frequently coprescribed in these patients. Acetaminophen and other analgesics may be metabolized differently in the elderly and need to be more closely monitored. For those patients who continue to experience disabling headaches and in whom risk stratification is low, triptans can be prescribed. Those patients with an intermediate level of risk require further cardiac evaluation. If stress testing is normal, then triptans may be prescribed. In any event, the physician should clearly document in the chart that the patient suffers from disabling migraines that have failed to respond to other therapies, that the risks and benefits were discussed with the patient, and that the patient believes that the benefits outweigh the risks. Patients in the high-risk category should not be prescribed triptans.

Our patient continues to have disabling migraines despite her advanced age. Her only known risk factor for CAD is mild hypercholesterolemia, which is well controlled with medication. Using a calculator to determine her Framingham risk (www.cardiology.org/tools/medcalc/fram/), we can determine that her estimate of a cardiovascular event is 1% over 5 years and 4% over 10 years. Our patient is therefore in the low-risk category and can continue to use her triptan. She will have documentation placed into her chart that she understands the risks and benefits as discussed above. She will continue to be followed closely at regular intervals; should new risk factors for cardiovascular or cerebrovascular disease develop or other medical conditions arise, her medication regimen may need to be adjusted.

KEY POINTS TO REMEMBER

- There is no evidence that age alone is a contraindication to triptan use.
- Routine screening with EKG and stress testing is costly and not sensitive in patients with asymptomatic CAD.

Continued

- For patients without known cardiovascular disease, base treatment recommendations on risk stratification from the Framingham Study.
- Low-risk patients can be prescribed triptans.
- High-risk patients should avoid triptans.
- Intermediate-risk patients need more focused cardiac evaluations with EKG and stress testing.

Further Reading

Dodick D, Lipton RB, Martin V. Consensus statement. Cardiovascular safety profile of triptans (5-HT1B/1D agonists) in the acute treatment of migraine. Headache 2004;44(5):414.

Loder E, Biondi D. Can this patient take a triptan? Review of the cardiovascular safety of the triptans and recommendations for patient selection and evaluation. Internet J Neurol 2004;3:1-15.

Prencipe M, Casini AR, Ferretti C, et al. Prevalence of headache in an elderly population: attack frequency, disability, and use of medication. J Neurol Neurosurg Psychiatry 2001;70(3):377-381.

Ward TN. Headache disorders in the elderly. Curr Treat Options Neurol 2002;4(5):403-408.

Index

Page numbers followed by f indicate figures and those followed by t indicate tables.

posttraumatic headache criteria,
136t, 137t

sinus headache criteria, 8, 9t

Intracranial hemorrhage

arteriovenous malformations and, 146

diagnosis of, 4

treatment, 146

Intracranial hypertension, idiopathic,
121–123

Intracranial hypotension, spontaneous,
41–45

Ischemic stroke. *See* Stroke

Isometheptene, for HIV infection
headaches, 117

Ketorolac

for emergency management, 99

for inpatient management of medication
overuse, 102

Language disturbance, aura and, 53t, 55

Late luteal phase dysphoric disorder
(LLDD), 75, 76

Legal issues, posttraumatic headache and,
135–139

Lesser occipital nerve, anesthetic blockade
of, 106–107, 106f

LLDD. *See* Late luteal phase dysphoric
disorder (LLDD)

Local anesthetic blockade

for nummular headache, 69

for occipital neuralgia, 105–107, 106f

Lumbar puncture

for cough headache, 66

opening pressure measurement, 41,
44, 121

Macropsia, 54

Magnesium, high dose, for menstrually
related migraine, 76

Magnesium, intravenous, for emergency
management, 99

Magnesium supplementation

for chronic daily headache, 114

for migraine treatment during
pregnancy, 85–86

Magnetic resonance angiography (MRA)

in carotid dissection, 30

in cerebral venous thrombosis, 4

in reversible cerebral vasoconstriction
syndromes (RCVS), 50, 50f

Magnetic resonance imaging (MRI)

in carotid dissection, 30

contrast-enhanced, in spontaneous
intracranial hypotension, 42f, 43

functional, in concussion
evaluation, 155

in giant cell arteritis, 26

in sinus headache, 7, 8–9, 8f

in spontaneous intracranial
hypotension, 43

white matter hyperintensities in,
12–15, 13f

Mass lesions, and transient neurological
symptoms, 48

Medication overuse headache (MOH),
79–83

emergency management of, 99

indications for inpatient treatment
of, 100t

inpatient management of, 99–103

outpatient management of, 81–83

over-the-counter medications and, 113

treatment failure and, 80–81

Medications. *See also* Acute medications;
Prophylactic agents; *names of
specific drugs*

client education on risks and benefits,
129–130

discontinuation of, inappropriate, 80

inappropriate or subtherapeutic, in
treatment failure, 80

overuse of. *See* Medication overuse
headache (MOH)

in pregnancy, safety of, 86–88, 86t, 87t

without coloring agents, 114

estrogen-containing medications
and, 75
migraine and, 75, 150
Subarachnoid hemorrhage (SAH)
aneurysmal, 4–5
familial incidence of, 5, 6
Substance allergies, 113
Sumatriptan, for emergency
management, 99
Superficial temporal artery, imaging of, in
giant cell arteritis, 26
Systemic vasculitis
affecting cerebral vessels, 49t
white matter hyperintensities and, 14

Temporal artery biopsy, in giant cell
arteritis, 24–25
Teratogen Information Service (TERIS),
medications, pregnancy risk categories
of, 87t
Testimony, legal, 138
TGA. *See* Transient global amnesia (TGA)
Thermal biofeedback, 114
Thrombocytosis, in giant cell arteritis,
24–25
Thunderclap headache, causes of, 4, 4t, 6
TIAs. *See* Transient ischemic attacks (TIAs)
Tinnitus, pulsatile, 121, 123
TN. *See* Trigeminal neuralgia (TN)
TNF-α (Tumor necrosis factor-α), 38
Topiramate
for hemicrania continua, 91
in HIV infection, 117
pregnancy and, 87
Transient global amnesia (TGA), 140–142
Transient ischemic attacks (TIAs)
patent foramen ovale and, 150
transient global amnesia and, 141
Traumatic injuries
of greater occipital nerve, and occipital
neuralgia, 105
of head. *See* Concussion; Posttraumatic
headache

legal issues and, 136, 138
of neck, and headache, 136, 137t
Treatment failure, reasons for, 80–81
Trigeminal neuralgia (TN), 93–97
clinical signs, 94
differential diagnosis, 94
nummular headache and, 68–69
secondary causes of, 94, 95t
surgical options for, 95–96
treatment, 95–96, 96t
Triptans
adverse effects of, 19, 19t
for childhood migraine, 18–19
daily use of, 83
in elderly patients, 158–161
for emergency management, 99
for menstrually related migraine, 75, 76
for migrainous vertigo, 61
nonresponse to, 110
pregnancy and, 87
serotonin syndrome and, 127–130
in transient global amnesia, 141–142
Tumor necrosis factor-α (TNF-α), and new
daily persistent headache, 38

U.S. Food and Drug Administration
(FDA), pregnancy risk categories of
medications, 86t
Ultrasonography, in giant cell arteritis, 26

Valproate sodium
drug interactions and, 102
in HIV infection, 117
for inpatient management of medication
overuse, 102
Valsalva maneuver headaches, 33–34, 64.
See also Cough headache; Exertional
headache
Vasculitis
central nervous system, 14, 49, 49t
cerebral, 49t
and headache, 47–51
systemic, 14, 49t